Edgar Cayce's
EVERYDAY
HEALTH

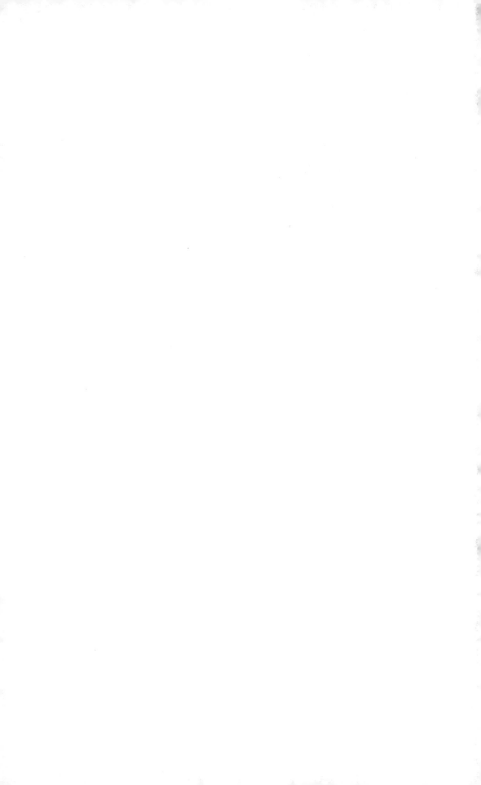

Edgar Cayce's
EVERYDAY
HEALTH
Holistic Tips, Remedies & Solutions

Carol A. Baraff

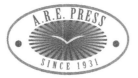

A.R.E. Press • Virginia Beach • Virginia

A.R.E. Press
215 67th Street
Virginia Beach, VA 23451-2061

ISBN 13: 978-0-87604-608-1

Disclaimer
The contents of this publication are intended for educational and informative use only. They are not to be considered directive nor as a guide to self-diagnosis or self-treatment. Before embarking on any therapeutic regimen, it is absolutely essential that you consult with and obtain the approval of your personal physician or health care provider.

Cover design by Christine Fulcher

Table of Contents

Author's Note and Acknowledgments ix

Dietary Matters
Collagen: The Glue That Holds Us Together 1
Olive Oil for Life! 4
Almonds, Beauty, and Long Life 6
Chocolate, Coffee, and Hold the Latte 9
Eating Our Way to Blood Sugar Balance 10
A Blueberry a Day 13
Fat: The Good, the Bad, and the Really Ugly—Part I 15
Fat: The Good, the Bad, and the Really Ugly—Part II 21
The Carbonation Question 26
Meat: to Eat? 32
A Toast to Wine 37

Health Aids and Strategies
Good Vibrations 41
Keeping Warm with Cayenne 43
Reconciling With Ragweed 45
Healing Lights 47
Castor Oil Creativity: The Abdominal Zone 52
Castor Oil Creativity: Head to Toe 56
Fruit Fasts for Fitness 59
Ipsab for Happy Gums 62
The Naked Truth about Sun Exposure 65
The Body Beautiful 68
Keg Therapy 70
Windows to Well-Being 73
Likable Glyco 75
An Atomidine Tale 77
The Best Exercise 79
Summer's Little Helpers 81
Water Cures 83
More Precious than Gold 87

The Silver Solution 90
The Remarkable RAP 92
That Revivifying Violet Ray 96
Feeling Good about Massage 99
Just Pack It! Part I 102
Just Pack It! Part II 105

Common Concerns and Disorders

Throat Coat, Be Gone! 109
Smoothing Scars 110
Correcting Constipation 113
Natural Help for Hearts under Pressure 115
Arresting Arthritis 117
Unseating Piles 120
The Joy of Holistic Childbearing 122
Sleeping WELL! 126
Healing Gout from the Inside Out! 129
Well-Soothed Soles 131
Sweetening the Stomach 135
Keeping the "Live" in Liver 139
No-Brainer Keys to Keeping Our Smarts 143
A Farewell to Ulcers 146
Kidney TLC 150
Keeping the Beat: Help for Skipping Hearts 154
Bringing Up Beautiful Babies 156
Putting a Stop to Stuttering 163
Taking the Punch out of Rheumatism and Neuritis 168
Damage Control for Cold Sores and Shingles 176
Hope for Hives 182

Holistic Perspectives

Healing Rocks 189
The Case of the Elusive Singing Lapis 192
Essential Oils: More than Just a Pretty Fragrance 196
Transforming Stress 199
Allergies: All in the Body-Mind 206

Hypochondria: When It IS All in the Mind 213
Closing the Door to Spirit Possession 218
Breathing as a Way of Life 224
Keys to Rejuvenescence 229
A Prescription for Healthy Living 234

Bibliography *239*

About the Author *243*

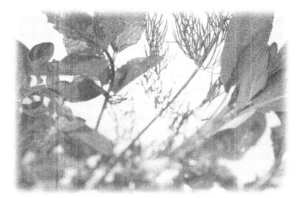

Author's Note and Acknowledgments

I f these chapters look familiar to some of you, it is because each one first appeared as an article in the Heritage Store's newsletter (Virginia Beach, VA) between the years 2004 and 2010. As a group they are a distillation of forty years of researching the Edgar Cayce readings and writing about their perspective on health topics, in particular. The monthly contributions have allowed me to present this amazing material in an accessible fashion and at the same time let the readings themselves have the last word. In some instances I have been able to go into more depth than ever before and to delve into some truly fascinating tangents.

I am especially grateful to Tom Johnson for giving me unprecedented free rein with topics, to my husband Jim Baraff for constantly reinforcing the thought form of a book, to Michael Reidy for being both fan and production angel, to MaryAnna Keller for providing faithful support and computer wizardry, and of course, to Edgar Cayce for continuing to inspire us all with a spiritually grounded vision of true health.

Please note: when you see this configuration {word} in a Cayce quote, it means that the author has supplied a word to make the reference more specific to her point.

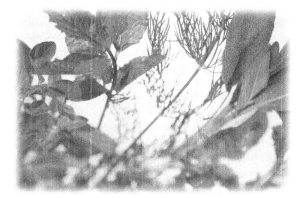

Dietary Matters

Collagen: The Glue That Holds Us Together

Remember the silly old song that goes "The old gray mare, she ain't what she used to be"? Now we can make a well-educated guess about that elderly nag's problem. Chances are she was losing her reserves of collagen—a term used to define both the multiple types of connective tissue that keep the body from dissolving into a shapeless mass and the protein-packed supplement found on store shelves.

Though the word collagen may be new to some, the substance itself has been part of our diets since our prehistoric forbears kissed their fruitarian diets goodbye. Meat and poultry are primary sources of collagen protein. It is in meat broths, in particular, (remember Mom's for-what-ails-you chicken soup?) that we encounter a highly nourishing form of collagen known as gelatin. Yes, those clear supplement capsules and the rainbow-colored undulating dessert that "there's always room for" come from the same source. Beside the Jell-O packages and the plain gelatin sold at most supermarkets, one can find gelatin mixtures for strengthening brittle nails—a use that's been recognized for over fifty years!

It turns out that gelatin—a sticky, rather tasteless powder typically derived from cow hides—is a super source of the two most abundant types of collagen in the human body: Types I and III. For those who have studied the Cayce material on diet and health, the mention of gelatin should ring some very large bells. A look at the readings on raw vegetables, in particular, reveals that at least one out of ten specifically recommend gelatin as an accompaniment:

> In building up the body with foods, preferably have a great deal of raw vegetables for this body, as lettuce, celery, carrots, watercress. All would be taken raw, with dressing, and oft with gelatin. These {vegetables} should be grated, or cut very fine, or even ground, but do preserve all of the juices with them when these are prepared in this manner in the gelatin.   5394-1

The readings seem to regard gelatin as a type of catalyst that helps the body to access or utilize nutrients from the diet:

> It isn't the vitamin content {in gelatin} but it is ability to work with the activities of the glands, causing the glands to take from that absorbed or digested the vitamins that would not be active if there is not sufficient gelatin in the body. See, there may be mixed with any chemical that which makes the rest of the system susceptible or able to call from the system that needed. It becomes then, as it were, "sensitive" to conditions. Without it there is not that sensitivity.   849-75

Gelatin's extraordinary catalyzing capacity, which seems to stem from its rich amino acid content, has been recognized for some time. As health writers James and Phyllis Balch point out: "The enzymes and hormones that catalyze and regulate all body processes are proteins. Proteins help to regulate the body's water balance and maintain the proper internal pH. They assist in the exchange of nutrients between the intercellular fluids and the tissues, blood, and lymph."[1]

---

[1] James F. Balch, and Phyllis A. Balch, *Prescription for Nutritional Healing* (New York: Avery Publishing Group, 1997), 34.

As we know, proteins are made up of chains of amino acids. The writers go on to remark, in an amazing echo of Cayce's statements: "Amino acids also enable vitamins and minerals to perform their jobs properly. Even if vitamins and minerals are absorbed and assimilated by the body, they cannot be effective unless the necessary amino acids are present."[2]

With gelatin valued so highly, the more easily assimilated hydrolyzed or "predigested" collagen protein seems like more of a very good thing. Created and patented by an American pharmacist in the early 1970s, this form of collagen has become available to the general public only recently. However, doctors, clinics, and hospitals have been using it for the last few decades in weight loss programs, healing of burns and wounds, joint and connective tissue support, and as a nutritional aid for the elderly and those with degenerative diseases.

As a hot new supplement on the retail scene, collagen protein is the latest "fountain of youth" with some basis in fact. Collagen of Types I and III is the most basic building block of our bones, ligaments, joints, tendons, muscles, blood vessels, and tissues. Type II collagen sources, such as glucosamine, MSM, and chondroitin, build cartilage, which is especially weak in arthritics because they don't produce it well. Another effective Type II source seems to be chicken cartilage soup! Recent studies with rheumatoid arthritis patients have shown a huge decrease in joint swelling and tenderness. In other research, chicken collagen helped to prevent attacks on healthy joints.[3] One is reminded of Cayce's recommendation to cook chicken well and then chew on the bones!

Besides serving as a special kind of internal cement, collagen is the primary building material of our skin, hair, and nails—all features that cosmetics have been invented to "improve." In aging bodies, the internal collagen manufacturing plant begins to slowly break down. If a lack of healthy collagen causes our appearance to slide, as evidenced by

---

[2]Ibid.

[3]Y. Toda, S. Takemura, T. Morimoto, and R. Ogawa, "Relationship between HLA-DRB1 genotypes and efficacy or oral type II collagen treatment using chicken cartilage soup in rheumatoid arthritis," *Nihon Rinsho Meneki Gakkai Kaishi* (February, 1997): 44–51.

wrinkles; thin, sagging skin; dull, brittle hair; easily broken nails, stiffening joints, poor muscle tone, and flab, then perhaps the right collagen supplement would help to keep that old gray mare kicking.

The benefits claimed for hydrolyzed collagen are so many, varied, and dramatic that it's impossible (and inadvisable) to list them all here. However, they include the best complexion of one's life; thicker, faster growing hair; hard, durable nails; more restful sleep, weight loss (when needed), relief of arthritis symptoms, improved muscle tone, faster healing of surgical wounds, and much more.

Some supplements include Vitamin C because its presence has been found to enhance collagen synthesis. Perhaps this would explain Cayce's preference for consuming gelatin with fresh raw vegetables, which naturally supply this vitamin.

If simply consuming gelatin is the method of choice, there are easy, and in some cases, delicious ways to make the plain powder go down. One is to sprinkle it directly on salads, using a shaker container that can be found in health food stores. A teaspoon or two over soup, perhaps along with a little parmesan cheese, is another easy option. The obvious healthy alternative is to make one's own fruit (or vegetable) juice gelatin concoction. Here's the basic recipe:

To one cup of juice in a saucepan on the stove add one tablespoon or one package of plain gelatin. Allow this mixture to soften for five or ten minutes. Then heat over a low flame, stirring often, until steam begins to rise and the gelatin has dissolved. Remove from heat, pour into a bowl, and stir in another cup of juice. Chunks of fruit (avoid fresh pineapple) or raw, shredded vegetables can be added if desired. Chill until firm. To make a more exotic and dessert-like whipped version using fruit juice only, chill until the mixture starts to thicken, whip in a blender, and return to the bowl for further chilling. It's a delightfully light finish to any meal and a welcome way to help keep us from becoming unglued at the same time!

Olive Oil for Life!

When it comes to citing the many health benefits of this versatile oil, both inside and out, the Cayce readings have plenty of company. In fact, of all the edible oils, olive oil seems to be the one that inspires the most agreement. New and time-honored uses abound in the kitchen, the massage room, and the personal care arena.

As a staple in Mediterranean diets, the venerable olive, along with the oil that is pressed from it, has a long history of use. Recently, some extremely encouraging studies linking olive oil consumption with certain health trends have emerged from that part of the world. Daily intake of this largely monounsaturated fat is now thought to play a major role in heart health by reducing both blood pressure and cholesterol.

The high value placed by the Cayce readings on olive oil is implicit in the literally thousands of times it was mentioned. Besides being the favored oil in salad dressings, it is often recommended to be taken internally as a mild elimination aid and "food" for the intestinal system. Regarded as beneficial for anyone, its purpose is to soothe and protect the intestinal wall.

Those who can tolerate, or enjoy, this oil's distinctive flavor should know that many readings advise taking it in larger amounts as a part of systematic cleanses, such as the apple diet and castor oil packs. In the doses recommended, which range from approximately two to six tablespoons, olive oil tends to purge the gall bladder, sometimes in a rather dramatic fashion. In the process, the liver, as the source of the bile that is stored and excreted by the gall bladder, is aided in its difficult detoxifying work.

Similar uses and doses are found in the recommendations of present day health advocates. In the finely tuned protocol of Dr. Richard Schulze, for example, olive oil is part of a blended daily drink that also includes freshly pressed juice, raw garlic cloves, and ginger. In the course of a five-day cleanse, the oil is gradually increased from one tablespoon to five.[4]

"Food as medicine" uses for olive oil may at times go far beyond internal cleansing. For instance, some cancer researchers believe that it

---

[4]Richard Schulze, *Healing Liver and Gallbladder Disease Naturally* (California: Natural Healing Publications, 2003), 42–43.

functions as a powerful disease preventive. Olive oil's protective effect is linked to its antioxidant properties and unique fatty acid content.[5]

Cayce's external recommendations are found in a huge variety of complexion, massage, and skin care preparations. One reading goes so far as to state that ". . . olive oil—properly prepared (hence pure olive oil should always be used)—is one of the most effective agents for stimulating muscular activity, or mucus-membrane activity, that may be applied to a body." (440-3) In the case of a woman with weakness and toxemia, nightly massages with olive oil were advised ". . . to relax and strengthen and feed the muscular conditions, and to bring about the better locomotion from the effects of the poisons as are being eliminated from the system, and to strengthen the body throughout." (5421-6)

Besides being recommended alone, olive oil is included in an assortment of massage formulas, such as an often-mentioned pairing with equal parts tincture of myrrh: "The myrrh, as an activative force with the oil, acts as a healing influence to the tendency of inflammation or drying of the texture or tendril effect of muscular activities of the system." (372-8) In this case the two ingredients are combined just before use to avoid spoilage, though this is not an issue with combinations of oils. Because of its gentleness, olive oil is also a natural in hair and body wash products such as "castile" soaps and shampoos.

The emergence of new and healthful uses for the timeless olive should come as no surprise. It seems fitting that there should be such a strong similarity between the words "olive" and "alive."

Almonds, Beauty, and Long Life

There can be no denying that the almond was Edgar Cayce's favorite nut (unless in a joking mood), although the reasons for this preference remain incompletely understood. Cayce's remarks on this tropical seed's nutritional content, cosmetic properties, and uses in preventive medicine have sent countless numbers running to their health food stores

---

[5]R.W. Owen et al., "Olive-Oil Consumption and Health: The Possible Role of Antioxidants," *The Lancet Oncology* (October 2000): 107-12.

and have probably been a major boost to the almond industry over the years. Now, confirmation of these benefits is beginning to come to light. In the nutritional arena, the readings regard almonds as valuable blood builders, stating: " . . . The almond carries more phosphorus and iron in a combination easily assimilated than any other nut." *(1131-2)* This nut is also recommended for its calcium content, and almond (or almond and hazelnut) milk is sometimes preferred to cow's milk.

According to USDA statistics, almonds are indeed high in phosphorus and supply 6% of the Daily Value (DV) for iron and 6% of the DV for calcium. Incidentally, they're even higher in magnesium (21%) and vitamin E (35%). Almond milk, which is widely available today, should be an excellent source of all these nutrients.

Along with hazelnuts (also a favorite) and other nuts, almonds are sometimes even regarded by Cayce as a meat substitute based on their protein and healthier fat content. The following comments are typical:

. . . Nuts are good, but do not combine same with meats. Let them take the place of same. Filberts *{hazelnuts}* and almonds are preferable in the nuts. 1151-2

. . . Those foods . . . have a tendency towards an alkaline reaction, but let the proteins be taken rather in the form of nuts and fruits—for the fats and oils, you see; these are much more preferable. 741-1

Almonds are so high in vitamin E and low in saturated fatty acids that some researchers have wondered whether they might play a role in reducing cholesterol. Sure enough, it has been found in studies that an almond-based diet significantly lowered total cholesterol and harmful LDL cholesterol and preserved helpful HDL cholesterol.[6] Other studies have shown that eating nuts, in general, will protect us from heart dis-

---

[6] Gene A. Spiller et al., "Nuts and Plasma Lipids: An Almond-Based Diet Lowers LDL-C while Preserving HDL-C," *Journal of the American College of Nutrition* (June 1998): 285–90.

ease.[7] In the most dramatic of these findings, in five large studies the risk of heart disease was reduced by a whopping 30 to 45% in those who ate nuts several times a week. [8]

In addition to health benefits, many readings regard the almond as a beautifier both inside and out. Cayce's skin emollient suggestions support the use of almond oil by the cosmetic industry for its legendary rejuvenating effect. Some refer to an almond cream or ". . . a lotion with an almond base." (1293-2) However, the most intriguing comments on this subject are of a dietary nature: "And know, if ye would take each day, through thy experience, two almonds, ye will never have skin blemishes . . . " (1206-13)

Other readings go much further, commenting that a few daily almonds will act as a cancer preventive. The familiar statement that "A person who eats two or three almonds each day need never fear cancer" (3180-3) is among the more general ones in the readings. A more colorful way of putting this follows:

> . . . and if an almond is taken each day, and kept up, you'll never have accumulation of tumors or such conditions through the body. An almond a day is much more in accord with keeping the doctor away, especially certain types of doctors, than apples. For the apple was the fall, not almond—the almond blossomed when everything else died. Remember this is life!   3180-3

The almond's possible role in cancer prevention has always been a puzzling one, but this is now being explored in animals. In a California study published in 2001, researchers investigated the effect of eating almonds, almond oil, and almond meal on colon cancer in rats. All were found to have preventive effects though the whole almonds were the

[7]P.M. Kris-Etherton et al., "Nuts and their Bioactive Constituents: Effects on Serum Lipids and Other Factors that Affect Disease Risk," *American Journal of Clinical Nutrition* (September 1999): 504–11.

[8]Paul Davis and Christine Iwahashi, "Whole Almonds and Almond Fractions Reduce Aberrant Crypt Foci in a Rat Model of Colon Carcinogenesis," *Cancer Letter* (April 2001): 27–33.

most effective of the three and surpassed the wheat bran and cellulose used in control groups. The authors of the study concluded that "almond consumption may reduce colon cancer risk and does so via at least one almond-associated lipid [fat] component."[9]

How much more encouragement do we need to eat our almonds?

Chocolate, Coffee, and Hold the Latte

When does something thought to be a health challenge become a health food? The short, skeptical answer is when it serves some group's interests. But with Cayce, of course, there is no such pat answer. Here's the scoop, and it won't be the same flavor for everyone.

Chocolate, or *Theobroma cacao*, is a kind of bitter bean that is native to warm climates such as those found in Mexico and Central America. It contains theobromine, a caffeine-like stimulant that enhances mellow feelings. This mood altering effect has been highly valued by cultures such as the Aztecs, who were extremely fond of a peppery, unsweetened chocolate drink known as the food of the gods. Now, research is showing that this assessment may not be so far off.

Consider the findings of Joseph Vinson, a Pennsylvania chemistry professor, who says that cocoa powder is a better protective antioxidant food than either green tea or garlic. According to his analysis, a 40 gram bar of milk chocolate contains 300 mg. of polyphenols, dark chocolate twice that amount, and cocoa powder 1,200 mg. In another study, Vinson and Harold Schmitz, a chemist at M&M Mars, found that cocoa contains the same types of proanthocyanins found in Pycnogenol, a complex antioxidant matrix.[10]

In the Cayce readings, however, chocolate receives only moderate praise. Ovaltine, a fortified cereal drink containing cocoa, is proposed as an alternative to coffee or tea in several cases. Several more readings

---

[9]F.B. Hu and M.J. Stampfer, "Nut Consumption and Risk of Coronary Heart Disease: A Review of Epidemiologic Evidence," *Current Atherosclerosis Reports* (November 1999): 204–9.

[10]Chris Kilham, "Coffee and Chocolate, the New Health Foods," *HerbalGram* 47 (Fall 1999): 21.

suggest cocoa itself as a beverage in small amounts. The ten or so references to chocolate itself are more ambiguous due to difficulties with overindulgence, cane sugar content, sugar and starch combinations, and digestibility. In other words, the ideal form would be free of starch and sugar and not overly sweet, so the Aztecs apparently got it right!

Coffee, or *Coffea spp*, is a rich, dark beverage made from a Middle Eastern bean that has been highly prized for centuries. The caffeine it contains (unless removed) seems to stimulate the dopamine pathway in the brain, leading to improved mood and alertness. Consumption is known to improve mental concentration, vigilance, and an overall sense that all is right with the world. According to studies by Vinson and others, coffee is also a top source of antioxidant polyphenols that can reduce oxidation of fats in the blood (a contributor to heart disease) by 30 percent.

The readings are perhaps unique in regarding coffee (or tea) as a nourishing food when taken black and a noxious digestive irritant when combined with milk or cream. In his twenty-five or more comments on this beverage, Cayce often observes that drinking coffee in moderation is beneficial, ". . . but for the food value and the proper strengthening the coffee should be taken without either cream or sugar." (829-1) Further explanation is occasionally offered: " . . . While the food values in the milk or cream may be considered of an equal value alone, when used together they form a condition in the lactic juices of the stomach itself that does not make for the proper eliminations carried on through the whole of the alimentary canal." (983-1)

There are those who feel that combining their coffee with some sort of dairy product (this goes for ice cream, too) is worth the intestinal toll, but we purists are not among them. We have learned to prefer ours black—but it isn't too bad with almond milk!

Eating Our Way to Blood Sugar Balance

Dietary fads are nothing new. In fact, there is more similarity than variety in mono-diets that limit food group choices for more than a few days. Compared to current fads like the Atkins diet, the Cayce approach with its emphasis on plenty of fresh produce, lighter protein sources, whole grain carbohydrates, and a minimum of sweets is a model of moderation. It is heartening to know that confirmation has actually been around for several years now in the form of the New York Times bestseller *The New Sugar Busters!*

In focusing on the "glycemic" or insulin–stimulating content of various foods, *The New Sugar Busters!* reveals an intimate relationship between dietary choices, blood sugar balance, weight maintenance, cholesterol, energy, and optimal wellness. Echoing statements found throughout the Cayce readings, this book may scare hordes of readers into eliminating refined carbohydrates, in particular, from their menu. And that would be a good thing.

Although it is targeted primarily at frustrated dieters and diabetics, *The New Sugar Busters!* speaks to a premise that is far more universal: Avoiding high–glycemic foods will prevent and even reverse the onset of a wide variety of chronic conditions, thereby adding precious years to our lives. In examining the soaring increase of sugar consumption in particular over the past 1,500 years, the authors comment:

> For hundreds of millennia, our ancestors ate only a low-glycemic diet. Back then, the pancreas was probably not called upon to secrete as much insulin in one day of an entire lifetime as it is called upon to secrete nearly every day of our modern post-infant lifetime! . . .
>
> We have had refined sugar only for a mere blink of time in humans' digestive evolution. Think about it—refined sugar and refined flour are "new foods". Is it any wonder that the incidence of diabetes and impaired glucose tolerance continues to get higher and higher? Maybe we eat too much sugar and simply wear out or exhaust our pancreas glands, which surely did not evolve to produce the quantities of insulin a typical modern diet demands.[11]

A careful search of the Cayce material shows that the link between

---

[11]H. Leighton Steward et al., *The New Sugar Busters!* (New York: Ballantine Books, 2003), 31–32.

sweets and pancreas stimulation is perceived quite clearly, although the terminology sometimes varies. A reading for a fifty-one-year-old woman who was overweight advised:

> . . . Little sugar, for this—as indicated, of course—makes for an activity upon the pancreas that, unless there is a great deal of physical exertion, creates the tendency for the increase of avoirdupois {weight} throughout the whole body itself.   1073-1

In the case of a twenty-six-year-old man with diabetic tendencies, Cayce commented: ". . . for when there is too much alcohol produced in the system, either by the addition of alcoholic stimulants or of the diet that produces the improper equilibrium of alcoholic condition, the pancreas and the liver suffer from same . . . " (4145-1)

The low-glycemic diet presented in *The New Sugar Busters!* has reportedly helped many people achieve permanent weight loss as well as the reversal of Type II diabetes. The authors emphasize:

> The only things you cannot eat on this diet are the carbohydrates that cause an intense insulin secretion. You must virtually eliminate white potatoes, white rice, bread from highly refined flour, corn products, beets, and of course all refined sugars, such as sucrose (table sugar), corn syrup, molasses, and honey. Also, sugared soft drinks and beer are not allowed.[12]

For purposes of comparison, here are some typical Cayce comments:

> Hence sweets or sugars from the sugar cane should be tabu. Use rather those that are of a vegetable or fruit nature, or the sweets that are contained in such.   795-4

> In the diet, beware of too much starches of *any* kind; that is, do *not* include . . . white bread or anything of this nature.   632-6

---

[12]Ibid., 8.

... Eat a good deal of potato peeling—that is, like the baked Irish potato—but not any quantity of the pulp.   703-1

As to those warnings concerning the pancreas condition—be mindful that in the diet there are not sugars taken, nor any of those properties that carry carbonated waters *or* any product of the hops, or of such natures.   2577-1

But when cereals or starches are taken, do not have the citrus fruit at the same meal . . . for such a combination in the system at the same time becomes *acid*-producing!   1484-1

Possibly the most important practical information found in *The New Sugar Busters!* comes in the form of a chart that provides the "glycemic index" for a wide variety of foods. Armed with this handy guide, dieters are empowered to choose their carbs with care rather than eliminate them entirely from the diet. The sample menus and recipes are helpful too.

In this time of increasing pressure to rely on "convenience" foods and questionable forms of dieting, finding the balance that truly meets our needs is more of a challenge than ever. However, the results are well worthwhile in quantity and quality of life.

A Blueberry a Day

Most of us will probably recall childhood berry-picking expeditions with pleasure—even if we did sometimes end up being chased by bees! At the time it was our taste buds that drove us outdoors to search for some of nature's more exotic sweets. Now it seems that the little morsels are good for us too.

Referring to berries in general as "nature's sugars," the Edgar Cayce readings recommended them for various reasons: to provide the diet with ". . . as much of iron as possible . . . " (4889-1), to " . . . not only . . . purify but clarify general conditions for the body" (1179-7), to serve as a food that is " . . . very high in the adding of B complex . . . " (3285-1), or to " . . . lend energy to nerve building forces and those that give to the blood force the eliminating properties . . . " (4730-1)

Statements such as these are fascinating enough, but when Cayce goes on to mention certain kinds of berries, the jam really thickens. Consider the following rather futuristic comment about blueberries found in reading 3118-1:

> In the diet—keep to those things that heal within and without . . . and especially use the garden blueberry. (This is a property which someone, some day, will use in its proper place!)

Exactly which healing properties the readings have in mind here are not known, but the health benefits of blueberries are definitely in the news these days. The discovery some years ago of truly stunning antioxidant properties has received the most publicity. In a study conducted by the US Department of Agriculture's Center for Aging at Tufts University of the antioxidant content of more than forty fruits and vegetables, blueberries soared above the rest.[13] This is important because antioxidants are believed to help slow the aging process by destroying free radicals produced during metabolism. Free radicals are responsible for cellular damage associated with cancer, heart disease, arthritis, and the aging process.

The study, which used aging rats as subjects, noted improvements in balance, coordination, and short-term memory. The daily dosage would be the human equivalent of about half a cup—an amount with an antioxidant punch of 1,771 International Units of Vitamin E (about sixty times the RDA) and 1270 milligrams of Vitamin C (more than twenty-one times the RDA.)

The primary antioxidants in blueberries and their close cousin, bilberries, are anthocyanins, the flavonoid compounds that give them their color. This means that while blue is good, bluer is better. So, as the neutraceutical importance of cultivated berries grows, it seems that the

---

[13]James A. Joseph et al., "Reversals of Age-Related Declines in Neuronal Signal Transduction, Cognitive, and Motor Behavioral Deficits with Blueberry, Spinach, or Strawberry Supplementation," *The Journal of Neuroscience* (September 15, 1999): 19 (18): 8114-121.

darker wild berries will retain the most antioxidant properties.

For those who need still more encouragement to head for the produce department or better yet, a sunny meadow, other studies point to many additional health benefits. These claim that blueberries are strongly anticarcinogenic, promote urinary tract health, improve eyesight, and may also assist in cases of arthritis, angina, and diarrhea.

With blueberries winning the healthy produce prize, what are its strongest contenders? Interestingly enough, second place goes to Cayce-recommended Concord grape juice, with about two-thirds the antioxidant activity, followed by garlic, kale, strawberries, and spinach. All are great ways to chase the doldrums away, but by far the best is to find one's own special source of scrumptious dark "blues."

Fat: The Good, the Bad, and the Really Ugly—Part I

Like spaghetti westerns, dietary fats tend to inspire delight, disdain, or both at the same time. We either hate to love them or love to hate them. This ambivalence is fueled by understandable confusion. Some diets avoid all fats like the plague, while others are virtuously low in fat and still others include surprisingly large amounts. Staples like milk, meat, and eggs keep swinging in and out of favor; the once-lauded hydrogenated oils are now evil trans-fats, and bad cholesterol is gaining acceptance as a disease.

While controversy may be stimulating food for thought, it doesn't digest so well. We need a place of harmony and balance for the fat in our food and in our flesh. The meal plans laid out in the Edgar Cayce readings have helped many to find this happy "middle" ground.

The best way to start is to look at the sources of fat in our diets. Very broadly, all are of either animal or vegetable origin. Most menu outlines found in the readings include items from both of these groups. Exceptions point to special, usually temporary, health considerations.

This installment will focus on animal fat. Cayce's preferred sources are certain types of dairy products, egg yolks, and fish oils. It goes without saying that these should be organic so that the nutritional benefits are not outweighed by the risks.

In the readings, milk in moderate amounts is generally regarded as a body builder and an easily digested food so long as it is not added to coffee or tea or combined with citrus juices at a meal. This is especially true for children and those who need to gain weight and stamina as part of their recovery:

> Now the body only needs rest, plenty of food . . . that digests well with the system. Milk, olive oil, and any condition that builds fat tissue in the system without taxing the digestive organism, or over-taxing liver or kidneys, see?   137-85

As that ideal weight is regained, the fat content in the milk can be reduced:

> Whole milk isn't always the best! It is best if you want to keep fat! That's what they give their pigs—usually! But keep down calories and too much of fats.   257-240

In many cases, buttermilk and yogurt (Bulgarian milk) are preferred for their digestibility and other intestinal benefits:

> Also we would add Yogurt in the diet as an active cleanser through the colon and intestinal system. This would be most beneficial, not only purifying the alimentary canal but adding the vital forces necessary to enable those portions of the system to function in the nearer normal manner.   1542-1

> . . . Milk—this in some manners is taboo for the body, yet in others is excellent. Those of the Bulgarian milk, or of the buttermilk would be the *better* for the system. This is acid in its reaction, to be sure, in *some* cases. Not so here! for the bacilli as is created in system through same will produce effects such that we will have a cleansed colon by the use of same.   5525-1

Cheese is more problematical as it is often high in fat and may not combine well with carbohydrates. However, the path of caution lies in moderate amounts:

. . . A great deal of fats will be hard on the body, as indicated by the lack of ability for digesting greases in the present. Butter fats and cheeses and such are well to be taken in moderation.

1409-9

Approval is also given to butter, advised in small amounts in numerous readings:

In the diets, keep away from fats of most any nature, though butter—to be sure—or milk, may be taken in moderation.   189-7

Mornings—citrus fruits with little else, unless brown toast and butter, or coffee and toast and butter, or rice cakes, or the like. 265-7

Some readings clearly propose butter as a substitute for meat fat when preparing various foods:

Coddled eggs, or prepared in any manner just so they are not fried in grease. Scrambled in butter would be very well . . .   306-3

. . . Do not have these {vegetables} cooked with pork of any kind! Most of the grease used with these should be butterfat, when they are cooked—see?   278-1

. . . No particles of grease {in beef juice}, other than butter in same.   261-20

This is not to say that butter is regarded as a perfect food for all. Trouble digesting fats with resulting skin rash means it's time to cut back at least temporarily and switch to vegetable oils:

. . . Not too much of grease of any nature, though butter—preferably those of the nut variety—may be used.   91-1

. . . {Corn cakes} when taken should be prepared in butter—or with the fats from vegetables rather than from the animal fat . . . 259-7

Eggs, included in hundreds of meal plans, are highly recommended with no expressed concerns as to their fat content. While the white portion is sometimes found to be overly acidic, the yolk is almost universally advised. Preparation methods mentioned include soft boiling, soft scrambling, and hard cooking. Use of meat fat here is a very definite no–no:

> Do not eat fried foods of any kind, *ever;* especially *not* fried
> eggs . . .   1586-1

Olive oil, salad dressing, and mayonnaise are all mentioned in connection with hard–cooked eggs. The yolk can even be a dressing ingredient:

> . . . Preferably use the *oil* dressings; as olive oil with paprika, or
> such combinations. Even egg may be included in same, prefer-
> ably the hard egg (that is the yolk) and it worked into the oil as a
> portion of the dressing.   935-1

An exceptional source of a beneficial kind of fat that is extremely high in vitamins A and D is found in the oil from certain kinds of fish. This may be one reason why so many readings prefer seafood to other forms of animal protein:

> In the diet, do keep body-building foods . . . Not too much of fats,
> but foods that are easily assimilated; plenty of fish, both canned
> and fresh. Doing these, we should bring the better conditions for
> this body.   3267-1

Some readings also focus on supplemental fish oils such as cod liver or halibut oil in liquid or tablet form:

> . . . the properties in the Cod Liver Oil or Halibut Oil or those
> things that give co-resistances in the vitamins that such carry into
> the body.   1278-6

. . . The use of those properties as will be found in that of the *fish*
oils, or of those that are mono-hydrated . . .   2654-2

. . . *We* would use . . . codliver oil . . . This is as of *sunlight* taken
into the gastric forces, of especially the duodenum.   501-1

Unlike most animal fats, which are highly saturated (more on this
later), fish oils are a highly unsaturated kind known as omega–3s. The
largest amounts of these unusual fatty acids are found in oily fish from
cold northern waters such as sardines, herring, mackerel, bluefish,
salmon, and albacore tuna.

According to holistic wellness advocate, Dr. Andrew Weil, omega–3s
are extremely important to health:

They appear to reduce inflammatory changes in the body, protect
against abnormal blood clotting, and, possibly, protect against
cancer and degenerative changes in cells and tissues. A great deal
of research suggests that optimal diets should include sources of
these hard-to-find compounds.[14]

In contrast, a hazardous form of fat is the grease or tallow from meat.
Although various types of meat are themselves often advised, so is keeping them lean in most cases:

. . . Eat little meats, and those that are taken should be of sinew
rather than fats . . .   3-1

And in the matter of the diet, keep away from too much grease or
too much of any foods cooked in quantities of grease—whether it
be the fat of hog, sheep, beef or fowl! But rather use the *lean* portions and those that will make for body-building forces throughout. Fish and fowl are the preferable meats. No raw meat, and
very little ever of hog meat. Only bacon.   303-11

---

[14]Andrew Weil, *Spontaneous Healing* (New York: Alfred A. Knopf, 1995), 143–44.

Clearly, the only good bacon (if that) is the kind where most of the fat is burned off:

> . . . to be sure, breakfast bacon may be taken if it is prepared very crisp without much of the fat or grease in same.   23-3

This same principle of leanness applies to juices and broths as well:

> Noon meals would be preferably the meat juices, rather than the broths—but little or no fat included in same when the juices are being taken from same.   13-2

It also rules out that old southern practice of greasing up perfectly good greens:

> Plenty of green vegetables but not cooked in fat; rather in their *own* juices.   25-6

> . . . Do not use bacon or fats in cooking the vegetables, for this body, for these tend to add to distresses in those directions of this segregation and breaking of cellular forces throughout the system.   303-11

If meat fats, especially of pork and beef, are bad for us, there is one thing that can make them even worse. The readings are categorically opposed to fried foods of all kinds, especially where meat fats are involved:

> . . . No fried meat, no fried foods at *any* time for the body. 461-1

> . . . Do not have fried food, such as steak or very fat roasts—they are detrimental to the better eliminations from the system. 675-1

> . . . No *red* meat; no fried meat nor fried food of any kind; not even *boiled* fat meat. But fish, fowl, lamb or the like may be taken.
>   978-1

As mentioned earlier, one way that fats vary is in their degree of saturation. Chemically, fats are made up of fatty acids—chains of carbon atoms with varying numbers of hydrogen atoms attached. The more plentiful hydrogen atoms become, the greater the saturation, so saturation levels can range from mono (one double bond in the chain) to poly (two or more double bonds). Highly saturated fats such as those found in beef pose a variety of threats to health, as Dr. Weil attests:

> Evidence for the health risks of saturated fat is overwhelming. In most people, a high percentage of saturated fat in the diet stimulates the liver to make LDL (bad) cholesterol in quantities greater than the body can remove from the circulation. The result is damage to arterial walls (atherosclerosis), impairment of the cardiovascular system, increased risk of premature death and disability from coronary heart disease, and reduction of healing capacity through restriction of blood flow.[15]

Dr. Weil considers beef fat the greatest threat to health. Cayce seems to have given that dubious honor to pork fat, followed by beef. In our little dietary Western, these are the really bad guys, especially when fried. For a healthier town, it's best to run them out of Dodge.

Fat: The Good, the Bad, and the Really Ugly—Part II

Our previous installment focused on dietary fats from animal sources. Using a spaghetti western analogy, we found that some of these characters mean well, others are probably not so great, and still others pose a danger to our long-term existence. Now that those little dogies have ambled off into the sunset, it's time to re-people our oater scenario with fats of vegetable origin. But vegetarians had better hold their horses before whooping it up. Good and bad fats abound in the plant kingdom as well, though it's the artificially engineered ones that are truly nasty.

---

[15]Ibid., 139-40.

Cayce's favorite oil is, of course, olive oil with occasional nods to wheat germ oil and peanut oil. This kind of fat is a good guy—the type just about anyone would want to invite to dinner at the rooming house:

Q. Would it be well to take a small quantity of olive oil daily?
A. Will be for most everyone, but well for this body.   2072-16

Because of its distinctive flavor, high quality (extra virgin) olive oil is most easily taken with meals and makes one of the best salad dressing ingredients around:

Q. Is it alright to take the olive oil and the yolk of the eggs as food?
A. It's very good. These may be taken on the green vegetables if it is preferable to the body, for the taste of the body, but these taken in small quantities are always food for the system.
Q. How much olive oil on a salad at a meal?
A. Teaspoonful.   846-1

If not including it with meals, another way to benefit from olive oil is to take it in tiny doses throughout the course of a day:

Very small doses of Olive Oil would be well to be taken. This should be taken often. Very small doses, meaning three to four drops to five drops at a time, not more than that. That is just enough to produce those activities in the gastric flow along throughout the aesophagus and through the upper portion of the stomach, so that the activities with same will make for the enliv-ening or a food to the walls of the digestive force and system itself.
                                                               843-1

Many health researchers now share the preference of the readings for olive oil, which was undoubtedly atypical at the time. Noted holistic health advocate Dr. Andrew Weil is lavish in his praise:

Olive oil appears to be the best and safest of all edible fats. The body seems to have an easier time handling its predominant fatty acid, oleic acid, than any other fatty acid. Replacing saturated fat in the diet with olive oil leads to a reduction of bad cholesterol (whereas replacement with polyunsaturated vegetable oils lowers good cholesterol as well) . . . Moreover, in populations that use olive oil as their main cooking fat, rates of cardiovascular disease are lower than expected for the amount of total fat consumed, and rates of degenerative diseases and cancer are also lower than in many other populations.[16]

A major reason for olive oil's safety is that it is monounsaturated. Although this is also true to some degree of peanut, canola, and avocado oils, Weil doesn't trust them for various reasons. And there have been no known comments from either source regarding grape seed oil, another Mediterranean favorite said to have cholesterol lowering and balancing properties.

Cayce's rare comments on peanut oil internally are in some cases even associated with olive oil:

Not good if taken by itself. If this is taken in combination with Olive Oil, or alternated, it would be very well.   1688-8

Some readings also advocate taking wheat germ oil for its high concentration of Vitamin E. While a diet rich in whole grains would ideally provide enough of this nutrient, in some cases a supplement is evidently needed to help strengthen the nerves, muscles, and reproductive system:

The vitamins that are needed, as indicated, are contained in . . . the Oil that will . . . produce a *better* regeneration of the activities of the system—it would be very good for everyone where there is a period close to the menopause, or adjustments of any nature— Germ Oil.   538-53

---

[16]Andrew Weil, *Spontaneous Healing* (New York: Alfred A. Knopf, 1995), 142.

Incidentally, there are a few sources of beneficial omega-3 fatty acids in the vegetable kingdom, though Cayce made no comments about them. They are the oils from flax seeds, hemp seeds, and a wild green known as purslane.

A highly regarded source of vegetable oils in the readings is certain kinds of nuts. The lighter, less oily nuts in particular are nutritional powerhouses providing vital elements in easily assimilated form when not overdone. Most importantly, along with other elements, they are a valuable source of energy:

> We would add to the diet these nuts, but not some of the others: filberts, almonds, pecans; black walnuts, we would add in moderation—not too much—but especially almonds and filberts. These will supply elements, with the changes wrought, to build back energies for this body.   3481-3

> . . . Nuts, fruits, whole wheat, and all of those that add *energy* to the blood and nerve supply.   65-1

Nuts are also easy on the digestive system, have blood building properties, and are an important source of minerals such as calcium, magnesium, and phosphorus:

> Let the diet be of those properties that bring stimulation, yet are easily digested . . . Those of the juices of vegetables, and of fruits and nuts, may be varied according to the needs of the system and as assimilation takes place.   94-1

> Let the diet be those that add building forces to system without giving too much strain on digestion. Rather the juices or broths from meat, than the meat itself. Do not use any pork or hog meat in any form. Rather vegetables, nuts, fruit. Do this in a consistent, persistent, manner. We will bring results and better conditions for this body.   192-1

> Let the diet be not of meats, as the basis or the greater portion of

a meal—but rather those of the vegetables, fruits and nuts, as build
both for the blood supply and the *minerals* of the system.   197-1

Well that sufficient calcium be taken . . . especially in nuts such as
the filberts and almonds and the like.   480-46

The oils and fiber found in nuts naturally aid the process of elimination as well:

. . . A small quantity of roughage, as of certain *kinds* of nuts,
would be well for the body; as almonds, filberts.   543-24

. . . This *(equalization in system)* we would find by taking those
properties in salts, as are created in fruits and in nuts themselves.
First these are active forces with the digestive system itself.
                                                                        108-2

The nuts receiving the most recommendations are almonds, with
filberts (hazelnuts) close behind. Comments on other varieties, such as
pecans, walnuts, Brazil nuts, and cashews, are usually positive, but there
are exceptions. Here is some typical advice:

. . . Beware of large quantities of nuts or nut oils, unless these are
almonds.   755-1

. . . Particularly have almonds, filberts and the like, more than
other characters. Of course, a good quality of pecan is well. But
the almonds and filberts are particularly good for the body.
                                                                     1861-10

One good way to eat nuts is chopped and added to a raw vegetable
or fruit salad. Nut butters and milks are the preferred forms in some
cases. It is important to keep in mind that nut oils are polyunsaturated,
meaning that they easily degrade when heated. Therefore, nuts are best
eaten when fresh and raw and should be kept cold when stored over a
period of time. Dr. Weil likes keeping a couple of nut oils (hazelnut and

walnut) in his refrigerator for use as flavorings in foods and regards small amounts as no great risk to health.

However, he takes a much dimmer view of polyunsaturated oils such as corn, soy, sesame, sunflower, and safflower (he refuses to consider cottonseed oil a food). When these oils are hardened (hydrogenated) for use in margarine, solid vegetable shortening, and their products, they become chemically saturated fats. But this isn't the worst of it.

Although polyunsaturated oils were once believed to lower choles-terol, they are chemically unstable and tend to react with oxygen to form toxic compounds that harm DNA and cellular membranes, "pro-moting cancer, inflammation, and degenerative changes in tissue."[17] All are extracted with heat and solvents that lead to the formation of dreaded toxic trans-fatty acids, or TFAs. Dr. Weil comments:

> I believe that TFAs in the diet damage the regulatory machinery of the body, significantly compromising the healing system. Remem-ber that TFAs are never found in nature, only in fats that have been subjected to unusual chemical and physical treatment. Some researchers refer to them as "funny fats," but there is nothing funny about what they may do to us.[18]

Now that's truly ugly. Who would have thought that a so-called chemical marvel could be worse than the villain in a hokey movie? On second thought, that's not so unusual, is it? Well, pardners, reckon it's time to call in the olive oil to clean up this town!

The Carbonation Question

Most of us enjoy at least occasional carbonation—that tongue-tick-ling, belch-inducing process that puts the pop in sodas, the "soft" in soft drinks, the fizz in spritzers, and the sparkle in adult beverages. But how does this small indulgence affect our health, and how much is too much

---

[17]Ibid., 141.
[18]Ibid.

of a possibly good thing? Uh-oh—turns out the question of whether to carbonate is one of those tricky INDIVIDUAL MATTERS where strong statements can be found to support both sides. A survey of Cayce readings and research findings, while providing some helpful answers, allows some of the mystery to remain.

Sparkling water, fizzy water, and seltzer are all names for the end result of carbonation—the process of dissolving carbon dioxide into plain water. This can, of course, also occur in nature, producing a sparkling mineral water with an upscale or curative cachet. The readings appear to refer to the artificially produced kind whether taken by itself, with plain water, in soft drinks, or in fruit juice spritzers (though the term had not yet been invented.)

Because carbon dioxide is a waste product of metabolism that is exhaled through the lungs, there has been understandable concern about overloading the body with an ostensibly toxic substance. So far, however, modest benefits and little harm have been found. In studies of calcium erosion in bones and teeth, carbonation itself was found to have a negligible effect, though sodas remain a major cause of tooth decay.

A small 2002 study reported in the *European Journal of Gastroenterology and Hepatology* found that carbonated water eases the symptoms of indigestion and constipation. The use of mineral water in these cases was believed to enhance the positive effects.[19]

Hydration testing has shown carbonated and plain water to be equally effective. However, some believe that carbonation may increase absorption of alcohol into the bloodstream and that esophageal irritation is also a possibility. And in cases of gastroparesis, a stomach disorder, carbonation can evidently worsen the symptoms.

A comparison with the readings shows more similarities than differences in these findings. Strangely, however, most of those that simply mention carbonated water or generalize about drinks that include it lean in a negative direction, while specified beverages are more often

---

[19]Rosario Cuomo et al., "Effects of Carbonated Water on Functional Dyspepsia and Constipation," *European Journal of Gastroenterology & Hepatology* (September 2002): 991–99.

approved. In the first category, thirty-one readings are basically positive on the subject (often with precautions about amounts), while another eighty advise complete avoidance, at least for the time being, such as during a course of treatments.

However, those that focus on cola drinks, other soft drinks, juice drinks, or seltzer are weighted differently, with thirty favoring carbonation, nine advising Coke without carbonation, and only five declining Coke in any form. These figures reflect Cayce's tactics in dealing with issues affecting the functions of digestion and elimination—if we can figure out how they apply and when.

In some cases the body's pH, or acid–alkaline balance, is clearly a central concern. In this context, carbonated drinks are broadly described as conducive to acid formation:

In the diet—keep away from fats, from any carbonated drinks or drinks made from carbonated waters. Do not take any of these, nor any of the malt drinks or things of that nature; nor vinegar nor anything of that nature. Keep close to the alkalines.   337-28

Eat right! That is, about twenty percent acid to eighty percent alkaline foods! Beware of all soft drinks, or carbonated waters, or distilled drinks of any character.   263-8

Q. Of what foods should I beware?
A. Those that are excessively acid-producing. Those that have been indicated of too much carbonated waters, or those foods that produce an excess of fermentation in their activity.   361-10

Similar concerns about certain types of alcohol show that this, too, was sometimes considered too acidic for the body to handle. Perhaps this is doubly true of alcohol and seltzer combinations:

Q. Is this trouble with the stomach a return of the old trouble?
A. Not so much a return as a continuation, excited by too much of carbonated or distilled waters, see? No hard drinks, no malts, nor any drinks of that kind for this body.   348-24

. . . Keep away from beer, wines, whiskey, or even drinks that carry carbonated water; or do so . . . to thine *own undoing!*

391-18

Q. Skin eruptions on back and arms? Cause and treatment.
A. Warnings have been indicated to the body of diets, especially as related to carbonated waters and hard drinks and hops in drinks. Eliminate these, this will disappear.   416-18

. . . Do not mix too much of varied characters of the carbonated waters with drink, or strong drink. These make for a disturbance to the very portions that are causing reactions.   877-16

Keep away from meats, wines, any form of drinks made with carbonated waters.   987-5

As mentioned above, skin eruptions can be a sign of toxic reactions taking place in the digestive system. Another person with eczema tendencies was told to: "Leave off too much of the carbonated waters, and drinks with same." (416-12) Similarly, in a case of acute rash caused by poison ivy, the advice was: "Little or no meat, and *none* of carbonated waters!" (1635-2)

Too much carbonation in the system can also be gas producing, as some readings attest:

As indicated, there should be the refraining from any carbonated waters, or those things that tend to make for gas in the digestive system.   1315-11

Take no form of carbonated waters, no form of *any* drink with those formations from hops or of fermentations.   477-2

Other comments were more generally negative with the reasons being somewhat difficult to interpret:

Do not take any form of drinks that carry carbonated waters. The gases of these, as well as all such, are detrimental and only add fire to the unbalanced chemical forces that are segregating themselves in the body.   1013-3

Do not take *any* drinks with carbonated waters, nor with the products of hops or the like. These are harmful, as they—through their activities upon the system—tend to charge this effluvium that has caused the disturbance in the circulation.   1709-6

. . . Never too much of any drinks with carbonated waters. These are detrimental to the better reactions of an already disturbed assimilation.   1772-2

. . . Especially *no carbonated* waters should *ever* be taken! These are hard upon the system.   1880-1

Underlying these prohibitions is the concept of carbonation as a stimulant that affects the body's chemical balance. In cases of intestinal issues, it can easily be overdone to the point of causing distress and even an allergic type of reaction. Carbonation should, therefore, probably be avoided in conditions such as digestive upset, acid stomach, poor assimilation, toxicity, and thinning walls.

With that covered, we can now turn to some of Cayce's more positive comments. The bulk of these by far concern Coca–Cola, which is regarded as highly alkaline! Taken medicinally, with or without carbonation, the beverage is regarded as a purifier of kidney, bladder, and liver circulation. Small, occasional doses are specified, and timing is important:

Q. Does Coca-Cola aid or deter?
A. Coca-Cola for the body is a stimulant, and will aid at times and deter at others. Taken when tired, very good, but do not gulp— drink slowly.   257-167

. . . If a few drinks of Coca-Cola or any super-alkaline-reacting vibrations would be taken, these would clarify and purify . . .
                                    1268-2

. . . This is one body that would do well to occasionally take a Coca-Cola; not to become as a habituate action, but occasionally this would be *good* for the body. There are influences in same that would purify the lower hepatic circulation, that would be beneficial. Preferably, though, use that perfectly prepared—*bottled,* rather than from the counter—for they are more uniform. 1334-2

. . . Or if desirable drink Coca-Cola—a little Coca-Cola; this will act almost in the same way and manner in purifying or clearing the ducts through the kidneys, and thus reduce the general forces and influences there.   540-11

. . . If the acidity is indicated through the kidneys, or from the urine itself, then drink a little of the carbonated waters, as would be indicated with Coca-Cola—but that which is *bottled* is the better . . .
                                                                540-11

Keep away from any carbonated waters, save at times—or rather regularly—we would have a little Coca-Cola. This, with some of the activities in same, acts upon the kidneys to aid in relieving the tensions there.   584-8

. . . *Carbonated* drinks may be taken, especially Coca-Cola or those of such derivatives. These will aid especially in purifying the activity and coordinating same through the kidneys and the eliminating system.   849-26

In these cases the carbonation itself is clearly regarded as a beneficial element. This is equally true with a number of other types of fizzy drinks, some of which might be prepared at home:

. . . Those drinks with a little charged water would be very well— as Coca-Cola or Orangeade or the like, if taken once or twice a day; for their reaction upon the system as related to especially the hepatic or the kidney *and* liver circulation would be good.
                                                                1476-2

Soft drinks such as Coca-Cola, Cherry Cola, Pepsi-Cola or any of the Cola drinks, may be taken in moderation, . . .   1945-1

Noons—we would drink a little Coca-Cola, Orangeade, Lemonade, or the like . . .   327-2

Then any mild drink such as half and half carbonated and plain water will be very well, or Coca-Cola would be very well, to assist in purifying the flow through the kidneys; but not until such improvement is shown . . .   2367-1

Coca-Cola, limeades and such are *well* for the body. These will act *with* the kidneys *in* the eliminations.   391-17

Coca-Cola taken occasionally will be helpful, but limes, limeades and watermelon, these add principally.   540-6

. . . When carbonated waters or drinks are taken, either Dr. Pepper's or Coca-Cola may be taken; but let such as these be rather as an extra drink and not too regularly—and of Soft Drinks *beware!*   487-22

Q. What drinks may the body have?
A. Any that agree with the body. Especially those that are half and half the carbonated waters, these are very good for the body; as ginger ale, or grape juice, or fresh grape juice. Any of these may be taken.   1055-1

. . . Such drinks as carbonated waters of ginger, as Ginger Ale, Coca-Cola, will be those to be taken by the body.   1210-4

Although it is hard to determine in some of these cases why the carbonation is approved, an interesting pattern emerges when comparing dates for all of the readings that mention Coca–Cola. Almost all of the pro–carbonation readings took place in the 1930s with spikes in 1936 and especially 1938. All but one of the anti–carbonation readings occurred during the 1940s. Whether this indicates a change in carbonation or soft drink production around 1940 may be impossible to determine now. But many other things changed during those war years, so why not soda pop?

How such distinctions might apply today is, of course, a very good question. Whereas Cayce sometimes preferred the uniformity of prepared beverages, quality and purity of ingredients may be greater issues now. Besides, it's fun to mix one's own drinks, always starting with some nice, pure water. Whether that water has a certain sparkle remains a highly individual decision that takes one's state of health into account.

Meat: to Eat?

With vegetarianism and veganism (no animal products at all) on the rise, this is probably a good time to revisit the matter of meat in the diet. As with many other issues, the Cayce readings take a solidly middle ground with strong qualifying positions expressed on matters such as times to refrain, appropriate amounts, preferred varieties, and methods of preparation.

The vast scope of this topic can be illustrated with some statistics. Many thousands of readings offer dietary advice, so it is not surprising to find that well over one thousand mention specific sources of meat such as lamb or mutton, ocean fish, fowl or chicken, and beef or beef juice. Crisp bacon, strangely enough, has over two hundred endorsements, wild game almost as many and tripe (ruminant intestine) over one hundred. Other delicacies advised at least from time to time include liver, goat, kid, pig knuckle, and blood pudding.

In other words, it is clear beyond a doubt that for most people under most circumstances the readings approve of eating meat (a broad term meant here to include fish.) At the same time, frequent advice regarding smaller portions is coupled with a relentless push toward healthier choices. The end result is a revised diet that supplies more vital nutrients while being lighter, less acidic, easier on the digestion, and better balanced.

Meat is an especially reliable source of protein, iron, and B vitamins, and many readings reflect this by advising it for its strengthening and nourishing properties:

Use or eat those foods that are body and blood building. Hence, once or twice a week we would have broiled liver, broiled fish . . .
                                                                              357-12

In the digestive system, and for the building in the system . . . it is necessary, with the conditions as at present exist, to meet these with sufficient of the vitim [vitamin] and of protein forces to create sufficient heat, and to give the supply of vitim [vitamin] to the blood through the hemoglobin constituent. More iron and vegetable forces. Meats, only those of sufficient quantity to meet the needs of system, never using hog meat of any character. Small quantities of beef, fowl and fish especially.   341-2

Fish, fowl, and lamb are typically regarded as the most digestible kinds of meat, although a strong, active system can certainly handle a little beef now and then. If the blood needs some extra nourishment, then it might be advisable to expand one's options:

Evenings—the whole vegetable dinners, which would include meat; and, at least three times each week, include among the meats those of calf's liver or of tripe—and pig knuckle. These may be altered, you see.   274-2

. . . Then we may combine those of a *little* meat, provided same is of the character that makes for blood building—as tripe, pig knuckle, liver, blood pudding, and such . . .   295-4

Wild game is also preferred in many cases for its superior nutritional content:

Eat what the body calls for; more proteins at first; never very much meat, unless game or wild meat of fowls and birds.   294-3

Pig knuckle is a rare exception to the ban on pork, which is usually either not mentioned or very specifically and emphatically to be avoided. This is presumably one of the main offenders in Cayce's repeated injunctions against eating "heavy meats." Another pork exception that apparently acts as a digestive stimulant for some is a little crisp bacon now and then—cooked long enough to get rid of the fat.

Regardless of the types of meat involved, the preparation methods most often endorsed are stewing, roasting, or broiling in their own juices. Deep frying is not advised under any circumstances nor is eating meat raw in most cases (sorry, rare beef lovers.) Thorough cooking is repeatedly advised and is the basis for Cayce's often misunderstood warnings against eating "red meat." Many have puzzled over this apparent color distinction in readings preferring lamb to beef when the real issue was probably one of digestibility. Warnings such as ". . . no red meat, either beef, mutton or fowl" (295-4) make this quite clear, as do the 257 readings, which repeatedly advise against rare beef in particular. The one exception found to this rule is a reading for a professional boxer suggesting that small easily stomached amounts of raw beef or beef blood be taken for strength, endurance, and energy.

This brings us to the health giving properties of concentrated juices created by thorough cooking of various kinds of meat. Beef juice is especially praised here, but so, to a lesser degree, are the juices and broths of mutton, chicken, and even liver and fish. Meat juice is regarded as strengthening, blood building, and body building to any system but is especially important for those who require liquid or semi-liquid diets:

> The *juice* of beef may be given as *strengthening*, but not the meat itself—no! Just the meat *juice*—not broth—but the *juice*, and *that* given in very small quantities. 154-1

> . . . Not much meat, but sufficient to give weight with the reaction in digestion, and enough to build on. Chicken broth is good, see? 147-30

Although all are beneficial, meat juices are carefully distinguished in the readings from broths, stews, and soups that are water based and much more diluted. Where a cup or more of the latter can easily be consumed in a sitting, a teaspoonful or two of the juice is just about right. One reading recommending pure meat juices notes that they can be derived from various sources, including beef, mutton, and liver. When asked about proper dosage, Cayce's response was:

> Sufficient to retain the strength and vitality . . . Tablespoonful of meat juice represents near about a pound of meat!   275-27

A simple recipe for making beef juice based on the readings is as follows: Cut one pound of lean round steak into half inch cubes. Place in a one quart Mason jar with the lid on loosely and set it upon a cloth in a saucepan of water. Simmer for two to three hours, adding more water to the pan as needed. Then thoroughly squeeze or press juice from meat and refrigerate, discarding the remains. Sip juice one teaspoonful at a time several times daily.

Anyone with digestive issues would do well to keep in mind that including juices and broths in the diet is a way of providing the nutritional benefits of meat without overtaxing the intestinal system:

> Let the diet be those that add building forces to system without giving too much strain on digestion. Rather the juices or broths from meat, than the meat itself.   192-1

A repeated precaution to observe when including any meat in the diet is to make sure it is as clean as possible and comes from a high quality source. Recurrent issues with E coli bacteria and other hazards make these warnings obvious.

Lest vegetarians, raw food proponents, and metaphysically minded folks become too alarmed by all this focus on meat, it must be noted that many readings do approve of meat-free meals, days, and even diets, at least for periods of time. However, if vegetarianism is to be embraced as a superior path, this usually means adding a lot more vegetables and fruit than most people are used to eating. Those with enough self awareness are advised to simply monitor their food cravings and include meat a couple of times a week, or whenever it seems to be needed. Ideas about eliminating meat in order to become more spiritual are shot down in short biblical order with the warning that this could do more harm than good:

> Q. Does meat affect one's spiritual understanding?
> A. If there is that consciousness in self that is affected. But rather, as the conditions, the experiences, the surroundings of each soul become spiritualized; for "It is not that which goeth into a man that defileth him but that which cometh out." But to attempt, where the bloodstream—where the body-building forces of the nature's warriors within self have been builded for generations, those that have required the stability or stamina of meat—to relieve self of same entirely is to take from the revivifying influences of that body. For, spirituality by the flesh is as the spiritual life in its essence, a growth.   443-6

In other words, removing meat from the diet too quickly could cause a drastic loss in energy and stamina. So although less reliance on animal protein just might be an evolutionary trend, or even an ideal, we blood type O's, in particular, sure need our daily protein, and it's hard to get enough from the vegetable world alone. Would anyone care for some organic beef juice?

A Toast to Wine

It should come as no surprise to learn that current findings on the health benefits of wine amply confirm Edgar Cayce's enthusiastic endorsement. Even the Concord grapes favored in the readings have been getting a lot of favorable press (pun!) lately. Those who delve into this material find that it's literally loaded with therapeutic uses for various kinds of alcohol. This is a strong position when one considers that most readings took place during and shortly after Prohibition!

Drinkable varieties make a rather large topic with recommendations for red wine alone numbering at least eighty. Approval for other grape beverages can also be found, as is evident in scattered references to white wine, champagne, brandy, sherry, and cordial. Proprietary tonics containing wine as an ingredient, such as Wyeth's Beef, Iron, and Wine, are endorsed in another sixty or so readings. Then there are the non-grape options, such as eggnog with spirits *frumenti* (apparently a grain-based distillation) or the occasional beer endorsed for its yeast content.

To separate therapeutic value from beverage associations, the readings encourage users of red wine, in particular, to treat it as a food with specific nutritional benefits:

> Wines and brandies are rather good . . . Wine, red wine, as a food rather than as a drink, is rather preferable for the body.   261-28

> Internal stimuli to the system of wine or champagne, or the like, will aid in centralizing the circulation, though this should not be too strong as to cause congestion in any portion.   264-25

> Stimulant is always needed where there is the tendency for the depressions. This will be helpful to the body . . . Wine—red wine— is sufficient.   264-47

> . . . Wine, if it is taken as a *food*, is good for the body—but never by itself nor just as a drink.   303-20

Although wine alone may be acceptable, most readings advise combining it with carbohydrates such as dark or whole grain bread or crackers:

> Red Wine, and not too sweet. Nor too much of it nor too often but this is very good—especially when starches are taken. 257-226

> . . . Small quantities each day of a red wine with black bread would be strengthening, and make for an alteration in the digestive forces here that will be the more helpful.   482-6

Taken in moderation, this combination is considered universally beneficial:

> *Wine* is good for all, if taken alone or with black or brown bread. Not with meats so much as with just bread. This may be taken

between meals, or as a meal; but not too much—and just once a
day. Red Wine only.   462-6

It is important to observe these guidelines as only whole grains carry
blood and health-building nutrients that are supplemental to those
found in the wine. Wheat, rye, and pumpernickel (check labels for whole
grain content) are all suitable sources:

. . . Also we find that a little (not much) Red Wine taken with
brown or sour bread (that is, black bread), or with Ry-Krisp or the
like, in the late afternoons will be well to add to the diet. About a
jigger or half a jigger at a time, this also sipped.   528-6

Wine is a food if taken with brown or black bread, or whole wheat
or rye bread.   365-4

Not when retiring; but about two ounces of red wine in the late
afternoon—with black or brown bread—would be very, *very* well.
It is strengthening, blood and body building. Let the bread, though,
be sour bread; preferably what is ordinarily known as "Jew bread."
                                                           340-31

Also, rather than any strong drink, there should be red wine taken
with bread; for it is a food. Not beer, not ale. Occasionally white
wine, or *red* wine; or the mixed—that are not heavy—are very
good. But red wine taken regularly with bread—black bread—is
good.   257-151

The readings make it clear that this combination is most beneficial
when treated as a meal in itself, meaning without the addition of other
foods (so sorry, cheese fans). The best time of day is late afternoon or in
the early evening shortly before dinner:

. . . Wine taken as a *food*, not as a drink. An ounce and a half to
two ounces of red wine in the afternoon, after the body has *worn*
itself out; that is, two, three, four o'clock in the afternoon—or cock-

tail time. Take it as a food, with brown bread. Not beer or ale, nor
any of the hard drinks—but *red wine!*   578-5

. . . Sips of the food values are the more strengthening. The red
wine should be rather as the meal once a day, with the black bread
only; preferably in the afternoon when greater strength is needed
and the reaction will be the better.   325-66

. . . *red wine* would be excellent if taken as a meal with black or
sour bread, in the evenings or late afternoon.   437-7

When serving as a digestive stimulant, the wine is best taken in
amounts of no more than an ounce or two at a time and then sipped
very slowly:

. . . Take with sour bread or *brown* bread at those periods when
there is needed the stimulation from the general activity of the
system; that is, at three, four to five o'clock in the afternoon is the
period when an ounce to an ounce and a half may be taken with
the bread and be beneficial.   404-6

The lighter wines or champagne should be *sipped,* as to make for
a settling of the stomach and to strengthen the body.   325-60

Though a dollop of wine may be a good constitutional for just about
everyone, there are definitely cases in the readings of overloaded systems where all stimulants need to be temporarily avoided. In the mean-
time, grape juice may be an acceptable substitute. There are also
precautions about avoiding hard liquor, sticking to the lighter wines, or
those with the lowest alcohol content, and making sure the body does
not become too dependent on alcohol.

In this day and age, when many people have allergic reactions to
sulfites added to wine and other foods, some prudent label reading is
also a very good idea. A host of excellent, even in-state, organic wines
that contain no added sulfites can be found today.

With these caveats in mind, it's an excellent time for a heartfelt toast—
to the mighty fruit of the vine and its fermented essence.

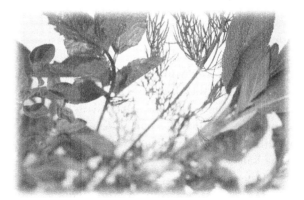

Health Aids and Strategies

Good Vibrations

Many folks today seem to be fascinated with the concept of vibration. Though the term literally refers to an oscillating or swinging motion, as in the vibration of the washing machine's spin cycle, the colloquial gist may bear a closer resemblance to a quality of energy or even to a feeling or generalized impression. Thus, a piece of music, a meditative chant, home, institution, workplace, or individual can all be said to have a particular "vibe." With the term so deeply embedded in our culture, it's not surprising to find an upsurge of interest in the health–giving properties of physical vibration. Here, as in many other areas, the Cayce information was ahead of its time.

In fact, over 375 readings recommend electric vibrator massages as a part of treatment in a wide variety of conditions. Here their primary purpose is to stimulate the superficial circulation in sluggish areas in order to help create a more balanced blood flow throughout the body. At the same time the slight but steady motion relaxes the muscles, relieves tension, and is ". . . excellent for quieting the nerve forces of the body . . . " (369-10), making this an extremely versatile form of therapy.

Vibrator massage works fine over clothing, broadening self-care—and home-care possibilities. However, using it over the skin following oil application apparently gives the circulation an even greater boost. This way "... the absorbing of the oil has a better distribution through the general muscular as well as regular circulation." (2452-2)

In one use of this type, the vibrator is used directly on the scalp after crude oil has been applied. Although a rub with the fingers may be a more typical practice, another effective option is "... using the electrically driven with the suction applicator" (4056-1) to work the oil thoroughly into the hair follicles.

A more usual site for electric vibrator treatments is the spine. A reading for a person with muscular problems due to injury commented:

> ... the vibration will act as the stimulation to those portions along the system, see, from the middle of the spine to the base of the brain—*deep!* It should be given ... along each side of the cerebrospinal system. This will make for a muscular relaxation and contraction that will make for the *adjustments* necessary ...
>
> 306-1

Similarly, a person with a partial dislocation or sprain was told:

> ... we only need to produce the vibration necessary to make the equalization of the nerve pressure through muscular forces over the system, and we will correct or bring the normal forces to this body ...   4101-1

The readings even view spinal application as a gentle way to stimulate sluggish elimination processes:

> The vibrations given in the electrically driven vibrator are to stimulate those centers (with this enlivening of the organs of the body, in the digestive and eliminating system) from the nerve plexus along the cerebro-spinal system, so that their activity produces nearer a normal impulse than is exercised by taking large quantities of cathartics ...   265-6

As with massage in general, vibrator treatments are regarded as es-

pecially helpful for the weak and the elderly, "to quiet the body at times
. . . " (326-12). The following instructions are typical:

> The use of the electrically driven vibrator should make for the re-
> laxing sufficiently for the body to fall to sleep. Use this over the
> cerebrospinal system, or around the back of the head, the neck,
> across the shoulders, even down to the lower portion of the body,
> as has been indicated.   728-2

Of course, the relaxation is greatest when someone else is conducting the massage, but that's not always possible, so investing in the type
of long-handled massager that can reach all the way down the spine
seems like an inspired idea. Good vibrations are closer at hand than
one might think!

Keeping Warm with Cayenne

Baby, it's cold outside . . . all right, only some of our winter so far has
fit that description. But north winds will blow, and it's important that
we know how to stay warm inside as well as out. There is a growing
awareness that one of the healthier forms of internal heating involves a
liberal use of cayenne or red pepper.

Capsicum frutescens, which grows wild in parts of the tropics, is closely
related to both the chili pepper and the sweet red bell pepper. It is the
primary ingredient in Tabasco sauce and is used extensively in Mexi-
can, Eastern Asian, Creole, and Cajun cuisine. In herbal medicine it is
typically employed as a general tonic and a specific for the circulatory
and digestive systems.

The Cayce material basically agrees with this usage, with over two
hundred readings referring to capsicum, capsici, or cayenne. While the
twenty-three references to cayenne focus primarily on its addition to
the diet, capsicum and capsici are more often employed as ingredients
in treatment protocols—keeping in mind, of course, that for Cayce food
is always medicine.

As remedies to be taken internally, capsicum and various forms of
capsici are regarded as " . . . a stimulant to digestion and the whole

body." (4454-1) Another reading giving more detail states:

> Capsici—acts as stimulation to the secretions, as the other forces
> are assimilated in the medicine chest (as it were) of the stomach,
> or through the duodenum and its activity upon the properties that
> are taken as food values into the system.   276-5

Cayenne is regarded as just as powerful externally. One individual
was advised:

> . . . A counter-irritant from the exterior forces will allow the circu-
> lation, both in the lymph and in the circulatory forces . . . to carry
> off and throw off more of the conditions. These, we would find,
> may be . . . any of the preparations whose *basic* force is of the
> cayenne nature . . .   488-2

Cayce's high opinion of cayenne receives enthusiastic support from
renowned herbalist Dr. Richard Schulze. An advocate of cayenne in both
internal and external formulas, Schulze believes categorically that:

> Cayenne is the greatest herbal aid to circulation and can be used
> on a regular basis. There is no other herb that stimulates the blood
> flow so rapidly, powerfully and completely. After all, no other herbs
> give you a red face—that's blood![20]

After explaining his belief (one very similar to Cayce's view) that all
disease is caused by some form of blockage, Schulze concludes that:
"Cayenne, without a doubt, is the best all-around, most powerful herbal
unblocker for maintaining your body's health."[21]

And how about pepper in the diet? Notably cayenne is strongly preferred by Cayce to other forms of pepper. Typical instructions are to use
it liberally to season items such as potatoes, stew, leafy vegetables,

---

[20]Richard Schulze, *Dr. Schulze's 2011 Herbal Product Catalog* (Marina Del Rey, CA: American Botanical Pharmacy, 2011), 92.

[21]Ibid.

chicken, and fish as the following excerpts show:

> . . . Potatoes, Irish potatoes, prepared with the jackets on. Best that these be boiled and then prepared with as much of the Cayenne pepper (no black pepper) as the body can take, with butter . . . and eaten in that manner . . . Fish may be used, but without the greases. Either that broiled in butter, or boiled or baked, and the seasoning of same should always have as much of the Cayenne peppers as the body can well take. No other spices. 4281-3

> . . . A little potato may be used in same [stew], and season quite highly with Cayenne or pod red pepper. Have this at least once a week.   340-44

> . . . Extracts of beef, prepared properly, with as much pepper (Cayenne) as can be taken for the system.   2553-7

Leave off all salt, or any stimulants such as seasonings of any kind, except Cayenne Pepper. Use this in the preparation of leafy vegetables, and in fowl or chicken.   5034-1

Ah . . . feeling those heat units yet? Perhaps it's time to hit the red hot pepper for warmer hands, feet, and heart this Valentine season.

Reconciling With Ragweed

Those who sniffle, sneeze, and swear their way through the annual hay fever season will probably be surprised to learn of this much-maligned herb's important health benefits. A member of the genus *Ambrosia* (Latin for "food of the gods"), ragweed is a North American plant whose flowers produce copious amounts of pollen. These tiny granules are capable of bringing even strong men to their knees from around the middle of August until the first frost in October or November. As a trigger of hay fever symptoms, including sneezing, dripping nose, and itchy, watery eyes, ragweed pollen ranks number one, hands down, throughout most of the United States.

The Cayce readings are notable in finding hope for the pollen sensitive in the ragweed plant itself, said to offer its own special homeopathic form of relief. Even more exciting is the suggestion that symptom reduction may be just the tip of the therapeutic iceberg. Most of the hundred-plus readings recommending "ambrosia weed" focused on its value as an internal cleanser and tonic for the liver and related organs. Since the liver is a major detoxifying organ, the theory is that a little TLC would make it that much more effective at knocking out those nasty allergens.

Those who consulted Cayce about their hay fever were advised to start making a tea with the young, tender leaves well before the plant began to flower. One reading put it this way:

Thus, we would find in this particular season, before there is the blossoming of same, the body should take quantities of this weed. Brew same, prepare, take internally and thus war or ward against the activity of this upon the body itself . . .

These will prevent, then, the recurrent conditions which have been and are a part of the experience of the body. This will enable the body to become immune because of the very action of this weed upon the digestive system, and the manner it will act with the assimilating body, too . . .

Begin and take it through the fifteen days of July and the whole of August, daily, half a teaspoonful each day.

Thus, we will find better eliminations, we will find better assimilation, we will find better distribution of the activities of foods in the body.   5347-1

As an internal cleanser, ragweed is consistently valued for its capacity to stimulate the entire gastrointestinal system without creating a dependency. More details are found in the following reading:

Will there be taken . . . in the system, at regular intervals, those properties that are not habit forming, neither are they effective towards creating the condition where cathartics are necessary for the activities through the alimentary canal—whether related to the colon or the jejunum, or ileum—yet these will change the vibrations in such a manner as to keep clarified the assimilations, and aid the pancreas, the spleen, the liver and hepatic circulation, in keeping a normal equilibrium. These [properties] would be found in those of the ambrosia weed . . . This will aid the digestive system, will aid the whole of the *eliminating* system.   454-1

Readings indicating a need for liver toning suggest a variety of substitute formulas for a ragweed and licorice laxative still on the market at the time called Simmons Liver Regulator. While some of the simpler versions contain only ragweed extract and grain alcohol, others include additional ingredients such as licorice, sarsaparilla, and tolu balsam. The following comments apply to a formula in the more basic category:

> . . . Where this *{Liver Regulator}* is given for anyone, the better preparation would be to make it out of the Ragweed, which is the basis of same . . .
> And you have better than Simmons Liver Regulator for activity on the liver! This for anyone! This is the *best* of the vegetable compounds for activities of the liver. Of course, if made commercially we would add some few other things to it.   369-12

Finally, another highly recommended use of ragweed is as a toner of the appendix through its capacity to " . . . stimulate the gastric flow not only through the liver and gall duct but to cleanse those areas about the caecum and appendix." (349-20) The readings regard this stimulating and cleansing effect as a powerful appendicitis preventive, stating: "If the most hated of the weeds were used {green} as a portion of the diet, it would never occur . . . " (644-1)

These are strong words of high praise for the lowly ambrosia weed, which could become one of our most loved if we gave it a chance.

Healing Lights

There's a great term for health-enhancing uses of light that hardly anyone seems to know. Heliotherapy, derived from the Greek word *helios* or sun, literally means the treatment of disease using sun baths. By Cayce's day, the heliotherapy options had expanded to include several different types of lamps that emitted parts of the sun's spectrum. Evidently it was quite common for health professionals, such as the eminent Dr. Harold Reilly, to use these lamps in their practice, and the readings include them in hundreds of treatments. Two of the three main types are at least somewhat familiar today. Fans of color therapy, take note—there are some interesting statements to ponder here.

Infrared lamps, with the most recommendations, have long been valued for their deep–heating and muscle–relaxing properties. Their rays lie just beyond the red end of the spectrum we can see and are longer than visible light. Unlike the infrared heat feature that comes with many massage appliances today, the lamps familiar to Cayce were quite large and were aimed at the body from at least a few feet away.

Referring to these emanations as *deep therapy*, many readings found them the perfect warm up for a spinal adjustment or massage, either before or afterwards:

> . . . (Use) the deep therapy, or the Infra-Red Light. This should be given after the deep manipulations—for these tend to relax and allow the activities of the blood supply through the disturbed areas; both the impulses of the circulation itself and the nerve flow.
>
> 920-11

> Just before the osteopathic manipulations are given, then, *relax* the body thoroughly . . . with the use of the Infra Red Rays. This should be the *deep* therapy . . . that is more inter-penetrating, that gives . . . the ability to prevent the improper . . . setting of tissue through all portions of the circulation. It will aid in those places where healing has not been accomplished, and yet make the proper corrections where tensions have been set up in the sacral and the lumbar area.
>
> 1083-3

The benefits of infrared light are truly deep if they extend all the way to the bones, or what Cayce referred to as structural portions of the body:

. . . Hence the deep therapy of the Infra Red should release these activities through structural portions as to build for a better, more stable, near normal circulation . . .   808-5

. . . {Use} as a stimulation for the deep therapy produced to the structural portions along the rib area especially.   2456-2

. . . The Infra Red is for the deeper application, or for the bone or structural portions of the body as related to their activity with assimilations and eliminations, while the ultra-violet works with deeper and the superficial, see?   443-4

As with the ultraviolet lamp mentioned above, using a plate of heavy green glass to modify the frequencies may also be advisable with infrared:

. . . use between the red ray and the body the green light or glass, that will take from that portion of the ray itself that which would be destructive to tissue that would replenish or rebuild . . .   338-1

The more unusual blue glass has a different function:

. . . use a blue glass between the body and the source of the light or the light itself. This would make for such an effect upon the tissue as to retard the tendencies for infectious reaction, because of the lack of coagulation and the removal by the flow of impulse of disintegrations from the energies of the body-exercise; and would also tend to make for healing forces.   1525-1

The ultraviolet light is also regarded as a form of deep therapy, though with superficial benefits as well. More properly known as a mercury vapor lamp, it has several different names in the readings, including ultraviolet ray and mercury quartz (or quartz mercury) light. Here electricity discharged through mercury vapor in a vacuum tube (mercury arc) emits a light that's rich in actinic and ultraviolet rays. Actinic rays, which consist of radiant energy, are found especially in the shorter light waves, and the ultraviolet are outside the visible spectrum at the violet end.

This lamp is not to be confused with the common sunlamp, which produces light in the ultraviolet spectrum as well. It is also quite different from a violet ray, a handheld device that emits static electricity when placed in contact with the skin.

Ultraviolet radiation is typically regarded as a circulation stimulant and infection fighter:

> Use the deep therapy of the ultra-violet that we have indicated from the first. Not too strong, as to destroy tissue, but of sufficient strength that there may be the reactions from the flow of the stimu- lated circulations to those portions of the body that *have* been affected by the tendencies for the accumulation of infectious forces . . . This will relax the body.   632-10

As with the infrared, it is helpful in some cases to use this lamp in concert with tiny internal doses of animated ash so the " . . . circulatory forces—that are aided by the releasing of the oxygen for the system through the Ash itself—may have the effect of the deeper therapy . . . " (901-1) Other readings (or sometimes the same ones) advise using " . . . the Ultra-violet with a green light {glass} between same and body . . . " (632-2)

When asked to explain the purpose of the green glass, Cayce responded:

> Breaks up the rays and rather than being of destructive natures, as it is in the destroying of tissue, it enlivens the good tissue and destroys the bad.   257-236

Blue glass might be of similar, or complementary, benefit to some, as in one reading advising the use of "spectro–chrome" therapy, or " . . . the ultra–violet ray broken up by the green and blue light {*glass*} . . . " (988-2)

Due to precautions respecting excess usage, ultraviolet light treat- ments must be carefully timed. Initial durations are often no more than a minute and a half to avoid burning the skin. Cayce also warned more than one enthusiast against conducting light treatments without the right expertise:

. . . None of these should be used except under one that has the training in such things—for this body as well as for anyone else!
                                                              480-16

Sun lamp, or the quartz mercury is the *better*—but under the supervision of one knowing, and not turned loose freely!   325-29

This leads us to the familiar sun lamp, another source of ultraviolet radiation that shares some benefits with both the mercury lamp and natural sunlight. Often referred to as the sunlight or carbon light, this was, in Cayce's day, an arc lamp that used a carbon rod. According to Cayce, "the Sun Lamp only stimulates the superficial circulation, or causes superficial irritation." (632–10)
However, this kind of stimulation can sometimes have therapeutic value when treatments are kept to a couple of minutes:

We would find it also well . . . that there is the *glow* from the Sun Lamp or Light on the cerebrospinal system—from the base of the brain to at least the middle of the dorsal area . . .   917-1

It will be found at times that the sun lamp will be beneficial. This does not mean to become merely rote, but the practical applications of heat—as the sun lamp—will be helpful.   1710-1

So far as this condition is concerned, it will be only when the body is tired or overstrained, overworked, that it would be of any particular benefit.   257-172

But the readings largely tend to view sun lamps as temporary substitutes for natural sunlight. As such, they are promptly discontinued when enough outdoor time can be had:

If there is *not* the exercise in the open air or sunshine, this is well.
                                                              257-240

From now on, or through a period until the body will be active sufficient, it will not be necessary; for the body can keep out of doors or in sunlight sufficient.   738-3

. . . As we find, the sun baths would be much preferable to a sun lamp in this particular season or time. These are the better violet ray at this particular time . . .   365-4

And this brings us back to *helios*, the sun, the original life-giving light. Here again, Cayce is very conservative about exposure, advising limited durations in the summertime before ten in the morning and after three or four in the afternoon. A good rule of thumb is to avoid the sun whenever your shadow is shorter than you are. When done properly, however, "sun bathing will add to those vitamins necessary, or aids the body materially in this." (275-27)

Castor Oil Creativity: The Abdominal Zone

One result of the Cayce information spreading far and wide is the emergence of a new kind of health nut, who will be known here as the castor oil convert. We probably all know at least one. When confronted with just about any of the ills that plague humankind, this person will reach for the castor oil, devise some often ingenious way of applying it, and then proceed to sing its praises. He's definitely on to something, based on the stories that are coming in.

The basic mechanics of castor packs are almost ridiculously simple. All that's required is a willingness to experiment with something truly messy. Since this can be an obstacle for those who prefer oil-free sheets, many castor converts were originally pushed into it somehow, whether by prayerful prompting, an opportunistic situation, or just plain desperation. They then developed a form and style that worked for them, perhaps unaware that the readings themselves encourage practitioners to make their own decisions about many of the details.

A prime example of this is the abdominal pack recommended in most of the seven hundred or so castor oil references. Here the choices, and sometimes also debates, start right away. To begin with, the pack itself consists of several layers of soft, absorbent fabric with some readings specifying heavy flannel and a few, wool. Users can take their choice of new material, old shirts, or pre-made packs, and even determine a pack's size and shape. While the ideal size in most cases is probably that of a standard heating pad, some readings imply that it might be smaller when targeting areas such as the liver. On the other hand, since extra sites such as the duodenum, colon, gall duct, uterus, and appendix are so often mentioned, covering the whole abdominal zone could be a very good idea.

With a pack selected or created, it's time to saturate it with oil. Although the readings tend to favor dipping the flannel in a pot of heated oil and then wringing it out, it's also quite easy to drip oil straight from the bottle onto a pack, thereby avoiding sticky kitchen messes. This also works well when replenishing pre-used packs, which is done as needed. A piece of plastic or handy oil resistant castor oil pack holder is always used as a covering to protect everything but the skin from the oil. A pack is easily warmed before and during use by an electric heating pad on a low setting. However, there are other ways to do this such as hot water bottles or hot salt packs.

Now it's time to decide how long at a time and how often a pack should be used. Pack durations in the readings vary from one or two hours to three or four or more, depending presumably on how urgently they are needed. A more organic method is to apply a pack at bedtime or at the start of a nap and remove it on waking, whenever that happens to be. Frequency of application in the readings ranges from once a week to at least once a day. For general toning purposes, hour-long packing three days in a row followed by a three- or four-day break is a good place to start.

Another important matter to consider is complementary treatment measures. Here we'll just take a look at other forms of cleansing, which are consistently advised following a series of two or more packs. One Cayce favorite is, of course, colon irrigation by means of enemas or colonics. Another is internal doses of olive oil, which range from a teaspoonful to a third of a cup, though a tablespoon or two is most typical. Other mild elimination aids, such as Castoria and Syrup of Figs, are also approved for this purpose. A rarer measure is castor oil itself, in doses that vary in size from one to four tablespoons:

Castor oil should be taken as an *eliminant* {as} . . . the system needs that of the excitement to the mucus coating of the duodenum, the activity of liver, and the reduction of the forces in the spleen's reaction with digestive forces, as well as the cleansing of the lower intestinal tract.   195-58

As an eliminant, very good eliminant! Necessary after taking such an eliminant that there be either Syrup of Figs or Castoria taken to *tone* the system without making a strain from the overacidity in the alimentary canal.   288-39

Evidently, this is only helpful in certain cases as other readings advised against internal dosage:

Q. Should the Castor Oil packs be continued, too?
A. Until there is the full reaction from the liver area, or so that the eliminating system adjusts itself, so that all poisons are eliminated from the system. These are better than taking it internally, see?
326-3

By now, it should be apparent, even to purists, that it's hard to find a wrong way to do a castor oil pack. So long as plenty of nice gooey warm oil is applied to the right general location, there will probably be some benefit. The underlying tissues will be softened, the liver stimulated, and the colon at least on its way to being cleansed:

We would increase the activity of the liver in its functioning, so as to bring about a better assimilation. We would increase this activity through that of counterirritation externally, using those of the castor oil packs for same, and these should be kept up until there is a full activity from same . . .   18-2

When necessary for the proper eliminations to be carried on in the system; nothing will be found better, for this aids the organs in their necessary overactivity in eliminating the character of drosses
. . .   325-43

. . . This will not only *relieve* the condition, but will enable the eliminating centers throughout this portion to throw off the refuse and prevent inflammation.   340-7

Healthier livers and nicely evacuated colons are always a plus for the entire digestive system and related organs. They provide extra space for our healing mechanisms to operate and are thus desirable goals. The Cayce material elaborates on this principle in some unusual ways that castor oil converts are sure to appreciate.

For instance, in at least one case we find a wraparound castor oil pack, applied front and back with low heat for an hour and a half at a time. Three consecutive days of this treatment are to be followed with a tablespoon of olive oil internally, and then later a two day series with more olive oil. It is noted that this will help to relieve tension and discomfort in the abdominal area.

A somewhat less novel approach is castor oil massage, also front and back in the instructions that follow. The friction provided by rubbing apparently creates enough heat for the oil to have its penetrating effect:

Begin with castor oil rubs (rather than packs). Take a very small quantity on the fingers and massage into the abdomen, lower portion of stomach proper, and across the lumbar and lower dorsal area. This would require patience and persistence on the part of those making the applications, for it would require at least two tablespoons full of the oil and at least twenty to thirty to forty minutes to do it; and should be done at least every other day. Massage into the body all that the body *will* assimilate, by gentle massaging.   266-2

The final step after a castor oil application is to remove excess oil from the skin. Some readings advise using a solution of baking soda and water for this purpose. A little soda sprinkled on a wet washcloth also works fine.

Finally, it's time to revel in the warm, fuzzy afterglow of a castor oil pack. The belly has never felt so soft! The entire body has seldom felt so relaxed! Maybe we'll hear of worship services at the church of the Palma

Christi next. After all, anointing with oil is an ancient spiritual tradition that remains with us today in the word, ointment: a soothing salve. Castor Oil converts, unite!

Castor Oil Creativity: Head to Toe

The previous installment focused on abdominal castor oil packs and some of the options that are available to the creatively inclined. Here we'll take a look at application sites other than the belly, a topic so full of possibilities that each castor oil user may have somewhat different needs as well as solutions.

This oil's uniquely penetrating properties have already been discussed. Perhaps even more remarkable is its capacity to promote absorption of irregularities on the skin's surface. Now absorption is a natural process in which disturbed tissue is softened to a point where the circulatory system can dispose of it by the usual channels. Castor oil application, therefore, enhances and supports the body's own efforts to heal.

Castor oil converts have really run with this concept with some spectacular results. That they have the backing of the Edgar Cayce readings is quite evident in the excerpts that follow, which take us on what is literally a head–to–toe cruise through the body. Note that the oil is probably most often to be used alone but can also be combined in interesting ways with substances such as baking soda. When in doubt, it's probably best to keep it simple and start with plain castor oil. Patience and persistence are definitely required here as some readings warn that obtaining the desired results can easily take a few weeks. So, here we go.

> Where there have been the accumulations from the lymph in portions of the body, as in face, these—as we find—may be absorbed through the system or they may be removed as they separate themselves . . . In absorption it would be well for these to be massaged with plain Castor Oil twice each day.   587-2

> Q. What can I do to eliminate the little bump on my forehead?

A. Use soda and Castor Oil, applied about twice a day—evenings when ready to retire, and morning upon arising.   462-16

The only addition would be that there be massaged over the broken abrasions on the body (as in the cheek, or lip): not over the places but around same, pure oil of the castor bean; or rectified castor oil. This we would do gently but firmly at least once each day, preferably upon retiring.   757-5

Q. What can be done for the sore on the ear?
A. Massage same with sweet *(olive)* oil or camphorated oil in the mornings, and with Castor Oil in the evenings; not to hurt, but just around the edges and over it.   650-2

Q. What should be done to eliminate the red spot on the nose?
A. This is not a blemish that will remain, but with the general system built up will gradually disappear. For local application, occasionally rub with *just* Castor Oil.   324-10

Q. One breast is smaller than the other; can something be done for that?
A. Massage—not the breasts themselves, but upon the *glands* that lead towards same—on either side, you see, and just between the two—with an equal combination of Olive Oil and Castor Oil. Do this each evening and we will make for the increase in such a way as to make rather the unison of the activity.   560-4

Q. Should both breasts be massaged?
A. Both should be massaged. The massage should be more on the *glands,* to be sure, *from* the breasts; than the breasts themselves; that is, about them and under the arm and downward, see?
                                                            560-6

Q. Should moles on the back be removed? If so, by whom and what method?
A. As we find, these are not to be disturbed to the extent of any

material or outside influence. The massaging of same (by self, or one who may do same for the body) with just the Castor Oil will prevent growth, and—if persistent with same (not bruising same)—will remove same entirely.   678-2

Q. What should be done for the small mole or soft growth on left side of back?
A. Use a small quantity of Castor Oil with a little soda mixed in same. This will make it sore for a day or two, then it will disappear!
Q. Just rub it on?
A. Just rub it on two or three days apart, for two or three times.
                                                                              4033-2

Q. What caused the birthmark on my baby's arm? How may this be removed?
A. By massaging it with an equal mixture of Olive Oil and Castor Oil it will be prevented from increasing. Marks on many bodies, as on this one, are for a purpose . . .   573-1

Q. What is cause of protruding bone on right arm near elbow?
A. A condition contracted some time ago by an injury there. Massage with Castor Oil and apply Castor Oil Packs {abdominal} each evening—this will relieve the tendencies for irritation.   556-18

Q. What happened when I stuck the pin in my wrist, that causes it to ache and pain me?
A. Bandage it about with a little Castor Oil.   1431-2

Q. What will remove callous or growth on right thumb?
A. As indicated, the care and attention is needed for the preservation. For the conditions that have grown, massage oft with Castor Oil—two or three times a day; and this does not mean once a day or once in three or four or five days!   257-202

Q. The small growth on the first finger of my right hand is still there. Should anything further be done?

A. This may be massaged with pure castor oil and be removed, see?   261-10

Q. How can I remove the knot on my right second finger?
A. Massage with Castor Oil *and* Soda—mixed.   303-32

Q. What causes the blemish on the left leg and what can be done to correct it?
A. This is a superficial reaction, and by the use of the Castor Oil rub may be reduced to very little indication. After this has been used for some weeks, just a little rubbed in each evening, then use Sweet Oil; this will change the whole reaction.   578-6

Q Anything I can do to take away knot on my ankle?
A. Massage with just Castor Oil, morning and evening.   308-8

. . . Massage the bunions or those portions of the pedals that disturb, with pure castor oil. The next day dampen plain bicarbonate of soda, or baking soda, with sufficient spirits of camphor to wet same, and massage this into the places that tend to be sore or callous. Keep up the treatment, and this will disappear.   365-2

Q. What is a cure for the hard and painful place under my right foot?
A. *Rest;* and using Castor Oil with Soda to massage same night and morning.   307-17

Hopefully this little tour has been both enjoyable and inspiring. Anyone who has ever tried rubbing castor oil into rough or dry skin areas knows how softening it can be. Move over, rejuvenating skin creams! Life's journey can be full of bumps, and castor oil is always here to help.

Fruit Fasts for Fitness

The phrase "food as medicine" applies perfectly to fruit fasts—limited duration diets consisting solely or primarily of fresh, raw fruit. This use of the word "fast" most likely comes to us from "steadfast," an apt term for the type of self-discipline needed by anyone on a diet. For some it may also imply "over quickly" as in lasting no longer than two to five days!

Regardless of whether one fasts for health reasons or as a prayerful observance, the central impact on the body is one of internal flushing and detoxification. Fruit, in particular, passes through the digestive tract very quickly and requires only minimal effort to process. This leaves energy to spare for other vital functions while the intestines enjoy their time off. It's actually a spa vacation because all that fruit fiber gives our intestinal walls a healthy and much-needed scrub. Picture driving through a tunnel before and after all the nasty accumulated grime is hosed from the walls, and you get the idea.

Cleansing these walls is good preventive medicine because it removes any impediments to smooth digestion, easy assimilation of nutrients, effortless evacuation of waste, and so forth. Cayce puts it this way:

> . . . the tendency for the accumulations through the colon . . . makes for some of the cells or pockets in same to at times carry for too great a period those fecal forces that become irritating and heavy.   843-2

> . . . There should be a warning to *all* bodies as to such conditions; for . . . would the assimilations and the eliminations . . . be kept nearer *normal* in the human family, the days might be extended to whatever period as was so desired; for the system is builded by the assimilations of that it takes within, and is able to bring resuscitation so long as the eliminations do not hinder.   311-4

Herbalist Dr. Richard Schulze echoes this view, and goes to great lengths to explain why "a constipated, swollen colon can cause an almost endless amount of seemingly unrelated diseases and problems."[22] With the gory details fresh in our minds, what are we waiting for? It's

---

[22]Richard Schulze, *Dr. Schulze's 2011 Herbal Product Catalog* (Marina Del Rey, CA: American Botanical Pharmacy, 2011), 28–29.

time to explore some fruit fasts.

The Famous Apple Diet

In this three-day diet, only raw apples are eaten. (Even under normal circumstances, the readings advise against combining raw apples with other foods.) The best varieties are Jonathan, Delicious, or any kind with bumps on the bottom though others will serve the purpose. No limit is placed on the number of apples consumed, though it is common to eat less each day as the appetite for this mono diet wanes! Drinking plenty of water is strongly advised. Minimal coffee or tea consumption is permitted so long as no milk, cream, or sweetener is added. The fast is concluded on the evening of the third day with two to four tablespoons of pure olive oil.

This elegantly conceived cleanse, which can be repeated as often as once a month, uses the abundant fiber and pectin found in raw apples to gently scour the intestinal walls. When the colon is at its cleanest, the large dose of olive oil provokes a sometimes rather strong reaction from the gall bladder and liver. Those who skip this step are, therefore, doing only half the diet! The readings comment:

> . . . This is to cleanse the activities of the liver, the kidneys, and the whole system—where there has been disturbance.   1850-3

> . . . And this would remove fecal matter that hasn't been removed for some time!   567-7

> . . . This is to change the activity through the whole alimentary canal.   3673-1

The Grape Diet

This three- or four-day diet consists only of large amounts of grapes—and plenty of drinking water. For this purpose the purple Concord variety is strongly preferred. Interestingly, many of the readings recommending this diet also advise abdominal poultices using the same type of grape. (A poultice consists of an inch thick layer of crushed grapes between pieces of gauze set over the belly and liver for about four hours.)

Although only scanty information on the purpose of this diet appears in the readings, the overall purpose seems to be general purification, and one reading clearly states: " . . . This will act as an aid in reducing those tendencies for gas." (2140-1)

We do know that the juice of Concord grapes is specifically advised for weight loss:

Simply drink three ounces of juice mixed with one ounce of plain water about half an hour before each meal: "To supply the sugars without gaining or making for greater weight." (457-8)

The Bananas and Buttermilk Diet

This is an oddball two- or three-day diet that is light, nourishing, and easily digested. The readings find it helpful in gently promoting coordination and internal cleansing without overtaxing the system:

> . . . The buttermilk and banana diet is rather as a balancing than as an eliminant: for it produces the absorption of certain toxic forces, and the adjustment of other conditions through the system.   538-65

A more moderate form of fruit fast is to simply eat fruit of all kinds for any breakfast or lunch. Sounds yummy—especially during the summer.

Ipsab for Happy Gums

Jokes about dentures, bridges, and root canals are not likely to amuse the huge number of Americans who suffer from some form of periodontal disease. In fact, this devastating condition—formerly termed pyorrhea—is the single most common cause of tooth loss after the age of thirty-five, and it's rising at an alarming rate. Symptoms range from tender, swollen, and bleeding gums to bacteria-laden pockets that eventually destroy the teeth.

How this works isn't pretty. Bacteria grow and multiply in the soft film that coats the teeth just hours after brushing. This film, called plaque, is composed of microscopic *S. mutans*, scavenging bacteria that cannot survive on fats and proteins but which view the typical high carbohydrate American diet as party food.

In the course of metabolizing these soft, overly processed foods, the bacteria leave behind an acidic residue that eats away at protective tooth enamel causing cavities to form. Eventually, both the interiors of affected teeth and the fibers that connect their roots to the supporting bone become corroded. Pus begins to form in the pockets, and the alveolar bones that form the tooth sockets become infected. As more bone is lost, the teeth gradually loosen, but unlike when we were eight, there's no tooth fairy to offer a reward.

Cayce's approach for around seventy individuals was to recommend a gum massage product known as Ipsab. Back when people were scratching their heads about the cause of periodontal disease, the readings attributed it to a particular bacillus, which in the presence of certain predisposing factors in the mouth is able to attack and weaken the gums. The breakdown of overly cooked foods was found to be especially harmful because it produces an acidic condition whereas the normal pH of the mouth is alkaline. Eating soft foods was also faulted as it leads to a lack of proper gum exercise and thus further lowers the resistance to bacterial attack.

Hence, Ipsab to the rescue! The unusual name was originally based on ingredient initials. The formula is a blend of prickly ash bark, salt, calcium chloride, peppermint, and iodine—ingredients with a history of use in mouth care. Prickly ash bark has been known as toothache bark in folk medicine. Salt helps to shrink the gum membranes between the teeth so the other ingredients can reach them more easily. Peppermint is often used as a breath freshener, and iodine is a recognized antiseptic.

It is hard to find a formula that is friendlier to the mouth. According to Cayce, using Ipsab as part of a regular oral hygiene program attacks the bacillus that causes gum disease while bolstering the natural defense mechanisms of the body. It also gives a helpful boost to tissue circulation and even improves the breath! Here are some sample comments on the methods and benefits of regular Ipsab use:

Once or twice a week. Apply a small quantity; or dip the finger into the solution, after it is shaken together, and massage the gums; or apply . . . to a tuft of cotton and massage inside and outside the gums, upper and lower. Where specific conditions in the teeth disturb, apply a small quantity on the end of a toothpick . . . and rub along the edge of the gums. This will be found most effective.   274-5

Using, then, for the teeth and gums, to strengthen same, those properties as found in that combination as has been given for such conditions through these forces.   257-11

. . . Do use Ipsab as a massage for the gums and it will make a great deal of difference with the teeth, the breath and the general activity.   3598-1

Having healthy gums is a wonderful thing. However, many readings go beyond this in claiming that Ipsab will improve the health of the entire mouth:

. . . with its application it'll *prevent* tooth decay, for it will cleanse the disorders that make for the reaction and keep the condition more alkalin in this area.   514-4

Some local attention is needed. The natural tendency of a distur- bance . . . is to make for a lack of the proper circulation through the gums and to the portions of the teeth themselves.
    If the solution known as Ipsab is used to massage the gums occasionally, it will make for a *strengthening* of the areas and a preserving of their usefulness. Once or twice a week this would be thoroughly massaged into the gums, and will make a great deal of change in the gums and the teeth . . .   987-1

This *[root canal work]* will be locally very good. But as we find, if there will be the suggested treatments followed for the *general* condition of the body, and a local application of those properties combined in the compound known as Ipsab—used as a massage, *much* of this condition with the teeth would be relieved without so *much* local attention. And we would find the mouth in much better condition for such work to be carried out, than in the immediate future.   1101-4

Putting so much effort into a healthier mouth may seem like a lot of trouble, but it's worth it. In the words of Edgar Cayce:

. . . It is by thy smile and not a word spoken, that the day may be made brighter for many a soul and in making the day brighter, even for a moment, ye have contributed to the whole world of affairs . . .   2794-3

The Naked Truth about Sun Exposure

Few topics polarize opinion like that of sun exposure and its effect on our skin. How much is beneficial—or harmful? Is tanning healthy? What about using sunscreen? Should we regard beach going as a health practice or a health risk? Both Cayce and some more recent sources bring essentially moderate positions to the hot debate.

A recurrent theme in the readings has to do with the health benefits of spending time in the open. Fresh air was considered so superior that even morning exercises were to take place out of doors, or at the very least, close to an open door or window. In addition to oxygenating the lungs, this activity is one way to expose the body to the natural ultra-violet spectrum needed by the skin to make "sunshine vitamin" D:

. . . It is the absorption of the ultra violet which gives strength and vitality to the nerves and muscular forces, which comes from the effect of the rays of the sun from the activities of the body.
                                                         3172-2

Today this vitamin seems increasingly important to health. Some surprising benefits have come to light in recent studies, which strongly suggest that absorption of vitamin D through sun exposure actually helps prevent some forms of cancer, such as malignant lymphoma and leukemia. Writing in *Parade Magazine* on June 19, 2005, Dr. Isadore Rosenfeld advises weighing the risks because too little time outdoors can be far worse than too much:

> Also, the further north you live in the U.S., the greater your chances of developing all kinds of cancer. Too little sunlight is said to result in a risk of death from cancer of the colon, prostate, breast or digestive tract 30 times greater than from sun-induced skin cancer.

These conclusions certainly sound like a strange reversal of prevailing views on the harmfulness of sunbathing. However, they're just a brief summation of results detailed at much great greater length in a *Virginian-Pilot* article that appeared on May 22, 2005. John Ott, pioneering author of the 1973 book *Health and Light: the Effects of Natural and Artificial Light on Man and Other Living Things*, finally has some company!

So, beach-goers unite—with ample precautions as to how long to bare the skin and the best times of day. At this writing, many doctors are agreed that in the absence of ultraviolet-blocking sunscreen there should be only minimal exposure, such as fifteen minutes a few times a week. While this may be appropriate for full sun at high noon, Cayce's longer exposures at non-peak times of day, with perhaps some indirect sunlight thrown in, seem much more workable. Here are some sample comments:

> Q. How long at a time should the body stay in the sun?
> A. For *this* body, thirty to sixty minutes would be sufficient. The exercises in the open would be *better* for the body *early* mornings, and late in the afternoon . . .   2-13

> . . . Never during those periods from 11:00 until 2:00. Then the body should not be in the sun, but the early periods and late periods are very well.   3172-2

Sunning in the early morning and late afternoon is not as conducive to tanning, but from the standpoint of vitamin D absorption that's probably for the best since skin coloration blocks ultraviolet:

> . . . *Do not* tan the body *too* much! That that gives the full activity to the capillaries, or to the exterior portions of the system, but too much sun is worse than too little; for light is penetrating of itself— see?   275-20

> . . . It is not so well that there be too much of the tan from the sun on the body. This forms on body to protect the body from same. Thus not so much of the tan but sufficient for the healthy activity of body.   3172-2

While visiting the beach, say before 10 a.m. or after 3 p.m., it's helpful to know that even exposure to salt water and sand can be therapeutic. As an accompaniment to sunning, many readings advise both ocean bathing and sand packs for their revitalizing effects:

> . . . Remain in sun and in sand after the salt bath or dip. Those sands as carry most of the curative forces in all minerals . . .
> 201-1

And when cold weather eventually returns, we may wish to keep in mind that SAD, or seasonal affective disorder, is caused by a shortage of sunlight, and the cure is a visit to a warmer place:

> Through the cold weather, or about the first of the year or sooner, we find that two to three to four weeks rest in a warmer climate would be very good for this body—the sun, the change in the climate, and the abilities to have more of the vital energies from the sun's rays would be beneficial for this body.   903-36

We "snowbirds" know what we're doing.

The Body Beautiful

Many Cayce aficionados will have heard of the Temple Beautiful, one of two legendary Egyptian sites of worship " . . . that *glorified* the activities of individuals, groups or masses, who had *cleansed* themselves for service." (294-148) This temple was reportedly built to inspire people through the power of aesthetic harmony—of its structure, the precious objects it contained, and the sacred activities it hosted. Since the readings also remind us to treat our bodies as temples, the comparison is obvious. Good maintenance will naturally enhance our best features, and the Cayce material overflows with helpful hints for giving that physical temple a healthy glow.

Where health is concerned, inner beauty is required for outer beauty to manifest. As the body's largest organ, our skin reflects how smoothly our "innards" are functioning as well as how it's coping with a host of environmental factors, such as variations in temperature, air quality, water quality, and an assortment of potential irritants. The digestive system, of course, does best with a balanced array of real foods, such as fresh fruits, veggies, whole grains, and light proteins. Refraining from junk food alone can clear up problem skin in a short period of time. The skin, hair, and nails often respond visibly to the addition of natural collagen sources, such as gelatin. Drinking ample amounts of water will have a hydrating effect on the tissues. Regular exercise stimulates both circulation and perspiration, thereby bringing healthy color to any complexion. Moderate sun exposure also puts the pink in one's cheeks along with other benefits.

Besides being an accurate indicator of how we're doing with diet and lifestyle, our complexion will always let us know how it feels about things we slather on it. The readings are a helpful source of information on substances that nourish the skin without being irritating. Simplicity is the key here.

When it comes to cleaning and moisturizing, our temples deserve the purest ingredients. Soaps made with vegetable oils are strongly preferred in statements such as:

Pure Castile {olive oil} soap is the better as a cleanser.   2072-6

> . . . a thorough cleansing with any good toilet soap, preferably that prepared with Olive Oil, or Coconut Oil rather than other characters of fats.   3051-3

Similar ingredients are favored in hair care:

> Use an Olive Oil shampoo. This as we find would be the better way.   1431-2

When prescribing for those with dry scalp tendencies, the readings take a different tack. Many include pine tar and petroleum products in the hair care routine:

> . . . have a thorough massage or shampoo with pure tar soap—at least once a week, and then . . . massage a little White Vaseline into the scalp after such a shampoo.   633-12

Pure crude oil and grain alcohol solutions are often added or substituted in treatments for eliminating flaking and improving texture and tone:

> Use crude oil, cleansing with a twenty percent solution of *grain* alcohol. Then massage just a small portion or quantity of White Vaseline into the scalp. This will cure *any* dandruff, unless it is produced—of course—by acne or some skin disorder.   850-2

> There has never been a better than the crude oil treatment. This would be given about two or three times a month, followed with a cleansing with a 20% solution of grain alcohol and then massaging White Vaseline into the scalp in such a manner as to leave the whole surface of the scalp not too greasy, but as sufficient into the scalp to produce the better application of whatever may be used. But this will grow hair on *most* bald heads . . .   636-1

When it comes to keeping the skin hydrated, several individual oils and many combinations can be found in the readings. Referred to as a

". . . food for the skin . . . " (1770-6), peanut oil is a substance that can
" . . . add to the beauty . . . " (1206-13) when used consistently:

> Use the Peanut Oil, as indicated, and we will find this will change
> the whole condition of the skin in a little while.   1770-7

Olive oil is held in equally high esteem:

> . . . Olive oil—properly prepared (hence pure olive oil should al-
> ways be used)—is one of the most effective agents for stimulating
> muscular activity, or mucus-membrane activity, that may be ap-
> plied to a body.   440-3

Soothing lanolin is a primary ingredient in numerous skin formulas.
Cocoa butter appears as a stimulating rub in readings for young children and pregnant women, in particular. Other complexion ingredients
sometimes mentioned include rosewater, glycerin, witch hazel, and pure
(not denatured) grain alcohol.

Here's an enticing combination. For a smooth complexion, work a
combination of peanut oil, olive oil, rosewater, and lanolin into the skin
after a warm bath:

> . . . {This} will aid in keeping the body beautiful; that is, {free from}
> any blemish of any nature.   1968-7

Time to start mixing, folks!

Keg Therapy

There are some unusual stories in the Cayce annals featuring a special type of inhalant: fumes from apple brandy stored in a charred oak
keg. One of these involves Edgar's wife, Gertrude, who reportedly used
this treatment during her recovery from an extremely serious case of
tuberculosis. Today, countless people continue to benefit from raising
their "spirits" with this unique form of inhalation therapy.

In Cayce's time brandy snifters (created to capture the fumes for enjoyment rather than health) were in common use, so inhalation itself was not as unusual as one might think. However, the readings were quick to recognize the potential benefits to the respiratory system of fumes from a particular type of brandy stored in a certain way.

A charred oak keg makes an extremely familiar looking container for the apple brandy base. Such kegs are used commercially in the storage of aging liquors because the charcoal absorbs impurities. One of these impurities is evidently acid from the distillation process, so while a keg might make the best kind of container in town, it's a good idea to rinse off the accumulated acids from time to time:

> . . . Rinse with *warm*—not hot but *warm* water, so that the accumulations from the distillation or evaporation of the properties are removed, and there is less of that influence or force which arises from the acids that come from such infusions.   1548-4

The readings are full of glowing comments about the benefits of this gigantic brandy snifter, which acts as an antiseptic for the lungs and other respiratory passages, with far-reaching benefits:

> . . . it acts as an antiseptic for all irritated areas; also giving activity to cellular force of the corpuscle itself. It acts as a stimuli to the circulation, then, recharging each cell as it passes through areas so affected by the radiation of the gases from this fluid itself.
>   3176-1

> . . . For the properties inhaled will work with the activity of the respiratory system, as well as the properties contained therein will act upon the influences of the liver and kidneys in their ability to be purified—in the assimilating of these forces that arise from the infusion of these influences indicated.   1557-1

> . . . This will act not only as an antiseptic, but will so change the lung tissue as to bring about healing of the lung tissues, and will also increase the abilities of assimilation, and we will have improvement.   5053-1

Keg therapy is recommended in over fifty readings involving a wide variety of respiratory conditions. They're enough to suggest that this treatment might well be beneficial for almost anyone.

If you decide to try the keg for yourself, the following pointers are a good place to start. For more detailed information you will need to ask a distributor or go straight to the readings themselves.

Gallon-sized kegs are on the pricey side but can last virtually forever. Be aware that a keg will be ready to hold liquid only after having gone through a full three-day water-logging process. This is important because good brandy is pricey too.

One keg will need two fifths or about fifty ounces of pure apple brandy, also sometimes labeled as Laird's 100% Captain Apple Jack (in Virginia), Straight Apple Brandy, or Bottled in Bond. "Applejack Brandy" is a less desirable blend that may be produced from a variety of fruit.

A filled keg should always be kept upright with cork inserted in a moderately warm place to encourage fumes to rise. (Avoid excessive heat and especially open flames!) When ready to use, simply uncork, insert a long plastic breathing tube, and inhale—cautiously at first so the body's reaction to the fumes can be gauged:

> . . . These will irritate at first, but use through the nostril for the stopping of cough, as well as inhaling into the lungs.   3594-1

Frequency and depth of inhalation can be gradually increased over time as tolerance grows. Watch for signs of too much inhalation, such as coughing and altered awareness:

> . . . Do not attempt to inhale too much in the beginning, or it will be inclined to produce too much intoxication for the body.
>
> 2448-1

In other words, let your comfort level be your guide. After a while you're apt to agree with Cayce, who advised:

> Keep the *keg*. This *is* as life itself.   1548-4

Perhaps some cool weather "keg" parties are in order with a BYOBT: Bring your own breathing tube!

Windows to Well-Being

The eyes have been poetically referred to as the "windows of the soul." Not surprisingly they can also serve as accurate indicators of our physical health. It, therefore, seems likely that a person's overall physical condition will be an important factor in how well the eyes, in particular, hold up.

A great deal is known about the complexity and sensitivity of the process by which images are transmitted to the brain. The eyes and associated structures are so delicate that a high incidence of assorted ailments is probably to be expected.

The link between eye disorders and certain types of health issues is well recognized. For instance, some eye and tear duct infections spread from sinus cavities in the nose. Conjunctivitis is often attributed to allergy. The herpes simplex virus can cause corneal ulceration. Infections of the inner eye are often associated with more systemic problems. Common disorders linked with aging include cataracts and glaucoma.

There are also instances where our eyes seem to function like canaries in a coal mine. Visual disorders may serve as early warnings of serious central nervous system imbalances, such as multiple sclerosis. Eye problems are also often associated with illnesses such as arteriosclerosis, vascular hypertension, diabetes, thyroid disease, and rheumatism.

The symptoms of eye disorders can range from mildly irritating to painful and debilitating. Fortunately, the Edgar Cayce readings offer a wealth of information on prevention and treatment of common complaints. Here we'll take a look at general health maintenance strategies, with a special focus on how they can help to keep our orbs clear and sparkling through life.

The foods we eat are just as important to eye health as to the system as a whole. Fiber and high quality nutrients are key ingredients here. Typical Cayce menus place a strong emphasis on alkaline foods such as vegetables and fruit accompanied by the usual whole grains, moderate dairy consumption, and light proteins. Gelatin apparently aids in the assimilation of vital nutrients from raw vegetables, in particular. The following excerpt gives some eye-opening details on the strengthening value of gelatin and carrots:

> But often use the raw vegetables which are prepared with gelatin. Use these at least three times each week. Those which grow more above the ground than those which grow below the ground. Do include, when these are prepared, carrots with that portion, especially close to the top. It *(that is, this part of the carrot)* may appear the harder and the less desirable but it carries the vital energies, stimulating the optic reactions between kidneys and the optics.   3051-6

The readings often link kidney and eye health, suggesting that the eyes tend to respond "sympathetically" to the condition of the kidneys. Tired, bleary eyes may therefore indicate that the body is dehydrated and the kidneys are not receiving enough fluids to do their job properly. The obvious solution is to clear the eyes by flushing the kidneys. This can be easily tested by observing the effect of drinking a glassful of water, a cup of watermelon seed tea, or a couple of ounces of Coca-Cola syrup in water. A fresh outlook on life may be the result.

Eye disorders can also go hand-in-hand with a variety of other common health challenges, including sluggish elimination, poor circulation, spinal misalignments, and infections. The premise here is that any or all of these imbalances will eventually impede the circulation to and from the eyes. In cases where the optic nerve had not been permanently damaged, Cayce would simply address the sources of each imbalance through treatments such as laxatives, herbal tonics, spinal adjustments, hydrotherapy, and massage. A lengthy series of such treatments might be needed for a noticeable effect on the eyes.

A well-known method for improving the eyesight, to which many can attest, is the Cayce head-and-neck exercise:

> . . . Take this regularly, not taking it sometimes and leaving off sometimes, but each morning and each evening take this exercise regularly for six months and we will see a great deal of difference.

Sitting erect, bend the head forward three times, to the back three times, to the right side three times, to the left side three times, and then circle the head each way three times. Don't hurry through it but take the time to do it. You will get results.   3549-1

These results can be truly "spectacular!"

Likable Glyco

From its pleasantly sweet medicinal bouquet and many helpful uses to its appetizingly pinkish hue, there is, indeed, a great deal to appreciate about Glyco–Thymoline. In fact, few Cayce medicine chest staples are as versatile as this soothing, alkaline fluid.

Originally promoted by its manufacturer for a variety of other purposes, Glyco has always been used primarily as a mouthwash, gargle, and spray for nasal and throat passages.

What's in this stuff? Ingredients include thymol, alcohol, glycerin, sodium borate, sodium benzoate, sodium bicarbonate, sodium salicylate, eucalyptol, menthol, pine oil, methyl salicylate, and carmine (an insect–based dye). It sounds pretty tame, but it's full of the kinds of herbs Cayce loved to advise.

When contacted in the 1970's, the manufacturer asserted that the Glyco formula had not changed since Cayce's day. However, the label was later changed to comply with FDA regulations, and today it is marketed simply as a mouthwash.

But would a mere mouthwash merit over eight hundred references in the Edgar Cayce readings? Not surprisingly, many recommendations have a few additional twists.

One reason for Cayce's enthusiasm is Glyco's alkalinity, which acts as a soothing, balancing balm on overly acidic mucous membranes. For this reason and probably more, a common recommendation for the intestinal system is to drink water to which a few drops of Glyco have been added.

Larger amounts are sometimes to be used in packs applied over various parts of the body including the eyes, sinuses, abdomen, and spine. In cases of tired, irritated eyes, a dilution, such as two parts of distilled water to one of Glyco, is common. This can be applied by means of an eye cup or a clean washcloth placed over the eyes.

Glyco's penetrating effect on congested sinuses is legendary. Here's what the readings have to say:

> We would use the Glyco-Thymoline packs over the nasal pas-sages, or sinus passages. Saturate three to four thicknesses of cotton cloth, or gauze, in warm Glyco-Thymoline, and apply over the passages, allowing such a pack to remain on for fifteen to twenty minutes at the time—and keep up until the passages are clear. Apply such packs whenever there is any distress—either in the sinus or in the digestive system. Such packs may also be ap-plied over the abdominal area to advantage, as well as over the face, see?   2794-2

A related recommendation is Glyco packs over certain areas of the spine using several thicknesses of cotton cloth saturated with the warm liquid for at least an hour at a time. One reading advises:

> . . . Apply heat over this, not too much but sufficient to cause these properties not only to relax the body but to be absorbed into those areas. Thus the osteopathic corrections, when administered the next day, will relieve these tensions and make for those ten-dencies towards a better coordination and a better alkalinity in the eliminations. Thus the activity to the kidneys will be aided, also the bladder and organs of pelvis, as well as the activity for the whole body.   3157-1

Glyco is also an indispensable part of Cayce's colonic recommenda-tions. As the readings put it: " . . . In the last water use Glyco–Thymoline . . . to purify the system, in the proportions of a tablespoonful to the quart of water." (1745-4)

Glyco–Thymoline is one of the few over–the–counter products that goes back to a time before the sleeping Cayce first uttered its name many, many decades ago. Clearly many of us still like our Glyco.

An Atomidine Tale

Many in the Virginia Beach community are undoubtedly already familiar with Atomidine, a clear golden liquid often used as a nutritional source of the mineral iodine (in minute amounts). Perhaps less well known is that this solution is said to provide the mineral in a uniquely bioavailable form. This is a good thing because iodine in its usual "molecular" state can be downright toxic whereas the "atomic" version found in Atomidine is apparently more readily utilized. According to Cayce, it's even less irritating than seaweed sources such as kelp!

Cayce is always one for unusual remedies, and the origin of this one is especially interesting. As the story goes, Atomidine has had several predecessors going back to the beginning of the 1900s or earlier. One was a thick black liquid used as a household remedy that was reportedly developed by an Indian shaman. In 1910 this was administered to a Dr. Sunker Bisey (B.C.), a Hindu scientist, chemist, and consulting engineer, who was a friend of Mahatma Gandhi.

Dr. Bisey was so impressed with the healing potential of this crude iodine compound in his own case that he subjected it to a thorough analysis. The eventual outcome was the marketing in England in 1913 of a relatively sophisticated product known as Beslin standing for best liquid iodine.

After relocating to the United States in 1917, Bisey established the American Beslin Corporation in the state of Delaware. As sales increased, the product was eventually distributed internationally. Later on, in 1926, it was sold to Laboratoire Durveaux, a New York corporation. After conducting clinical studies and collecting medical data and product testimonials, this company expanded the use of Beslin to liquid and ointment form and began promoting it in the fields of dentistry and veterinary medicine.

In 1931 Dr. Bisey, then sixty-four years of age, traveled to Virginia Beach to consult with Edgar Cayce about Atomidine as his product had come to be called. The readings had long indicated that iodine would be almost universally beneficial to health if it could somehow be rendered less toxic.

Cayce found the formula satisfactory but recommended some

changes in preparation that would bring more uniform results. Bisey performed some experiments, received several subsequent readings, and was aided financially by a man named Lester Hofheimer, who funded hospital research in various parts of the country.

Following Bisey's death in 1935, other family members continued to manage the business with Shieffelin and Company of New York acting as manufacturer. Sales gradually diminished over the next several decades due to the advent of the new "wonder drugs." In an effort to preserve the formula and keep Atomidine available, the Heritage Store in Virginia Beach acquired the manufacturing and distribution rights in 1974.[23]

In the Cayce readings Atomidine is mentioned well over eight hundred times. While never regarding it as a cure-all, the readings do observe that due to a common tendency to develop excess potash or potassium in the system, there are few human ailments that will not respond positively to the iodine's balancing influence when used correctly. This suggests that Atomidine can be considered a specific for imbalances in the glandular and intestinal systems. Properly diluted, it also makes an excellent gargle for tender throats and an antiseptic for skin abrasions.

There is much more that might be added regarding usage, but the focus here will be on precautions. Since a single drop of Atomidine supplies four times the minimum daily requirement of iodine, users are strongly advised to start small. This means beginning a dosage cycle (check the readings for examples) with no more than one drop daily and possibly less. To create a smaller dose, simply stir one drop into half a glass of water and then pour half of that down the drain. Atomidine is always contraindicated while other sources of iodine (kelp, kelp salt, multivitamins) are being taken and should never be used by those with heart problems. Too much iodine can cause nervousness, insomnia, skin rash, and rapid heartbeat, but when the amount is just right, energy simply soars!

---

[23]Carol A. Baraff, *The Atomidine Story* (Virginia: Heritage Publications, 1978), 1–2.

The Best Exercise

Nowhere is the term "Use it or lose it" more apropos than in matters of physical fitness. Trim, flexible, well-contoured bodies are, by definition, bodies in motion. Sedentary habits quickly give rise to less complimentary adjectives. More importantly, the exterior reflects what's going on inside, and exercise has far-reaching benefits for circulation, muscles, nerves, and more.

Although the best exercises for us must (sometimes by default) be defined as those we actually do, more specific parameters are found in the Cayce readings and in a highly recommended book, *The Edgar Cayce Handbook for Health Through Drugless Therapy* by master therapist Harold J. Reilly and Ruth Hagy Brod.

One thing we learn is that certain exercises are best for us at certain times of day. For instance, "setting up" exercises, in which the arms are swung and circled and the upper torso rotated, were typically suggested first thing in the morning. One reading comments that " . . . this will bring strength to the lungs, vitality to the blood supply, and a new life, as it were, to the muscular forces of the body." (4462-1)

Morning calisthenics may also include rising on the toes and stretching the arms high over the head while breathing in and then swinging them back and lowering them slowly while breathing out. " . . . This is an excellent exercise for posture and for aiding in keeping this balance . . . " (1773-1)

A type of routine that includes stretching, bending from the waist, and the well-known head and neck exercises, in which the neck is gently stretched in each direction and then rotated both ways, is recommended for " . . . giving a better circulation through the whole area from the abdomen, through the diaphragm, through the lungs, head and neck." (470-37)

The stretching and bending motion, in particular, (in this case morning and evening) is considered a specific for hemorrhoids with the claim that " . . . if this is taken regularly these will disappear—of themselves!" (2823-2)

A typical Cayce guideline for choosing a program based on time of day is vertical calisthenics in the morning consisting of " . . . circular motion of hands and upper portion of body" and horizontal ones for the legs and lower torso in the evening: " . . . exercises for the blood flow away from head . . . " "Swinging, circular motion then of lower portion of body . . . " (288-11) The exceptions to this rule seem to be cat stretches and walking.

Exercises that imitate the arching back and extended limbs of the cat are so highly regarded that Cayce states categorically, " . . . No better exercises may be taken than . . . the cat–stretching exercises." (681-2) Walking is almost universally endorsed when properly done:

Walking is the best exercise, but don't take this spasmodically. Have a regular time and do it, rain or shine!   1968-9

. . . Walking is the best exercise, but this—though—in the *open* when at all practical.   1530-2

. . . Walking is one of the *best* of exercises; walking, swimming, *anything* that has the calisthenics; tennis, handball, badminton; *any* of these activities for the body.   2153-4

This focus on the health benefits of walking and other types of exercise has received recent confirmation from several long-term studies. One, based on records made during the well-known Framingham Heart Study, concluded that even waiting until age fifty to start a "very active" exercise program significantly improved heart health and increased life expectancy by up to three and a half years.[24] Another examining close to five hundred adults found that cardiovascular fitness was improved by only half an hour of moderate to brisk walking at least three times a week.[25] A third study, which followed nearly forty thousand healthy women over several years, concluded that those who regularly walked at least one hour a week reduced their risk of coronary heart disease by half.[26]

---

[24]Fredrick M. Wigley, "Exercise after 50 Can Add Three Years to Life Expectancy," *Duke Medicine Health News* (January 2006): 2.

[25]Ibid.

[26]S. Mora et al., "Association of Physical Activity and Body Mass Index with Novel and Traditional Cardiovascular Biomarkers in Women," *Journal of the American Medical Association* (March 2006): 1412-19.

Finding the right exercise program is an individual matter which takes experimentation to get it right. One clue is that the body will feel deeply relaxed and vitally energized at the same time:

It's well that each body, every body, take exercise to counteract the daily routine activity, so as to produce rest.   416-3

The best way to acquire the correct amount of pep is to take the exercise!   288-38

Yes, it's true. Fitness simply feels better.

Summer's Little Helpers

Fellow outdoor lovers, rejoice! It's always so liberating to throw off the outerwear and expose that overly swaddled body to the elements. But wait—how to make the most of all that lovely fresh air and sunshine without overdoing it? Fortunately, the Cayce readings abound in helpful hints and home remedies designed to help us make the summer months as healthy and comfortable as possible.

Injunctions to regularly spend time in nature are found throughout the readings. Breathing the oxygenated air, absorbing the rays, listening to the birdsong, smelling the flowers, gazing at sunsets—all are considered highly beneficial at body, mind, and soul levels. Exercise is usually to be performed outdoors or at the very least, before an open window. Summer naturally lends itself to walks, swims, bike rides, skating, sports, and games of many kinds. But readings for folks unable to exercise also advise outdoor time, even when it takes the form of a siesta!

Although it's hard to breathe in too much air, there are, of course, many common outdoor hazards, such as dehydration, heat rash, insect bites, poison ivy, allergens, sore muscles, and overexposure to the elements. That's where the helpful hints come in.

The no-brainer ways to stay properly hydrated are to avoid excess sun and heat exposure and to drink plenty of non-alcoholic liquids. However, dehydration seems to be quite common, perhaps because it is easy to underestimate the amount of body fluid lost through perspiration. Because the skin is a major organ of elimination, the readings regard a daily sweat as vital to health. Antiperspirants are therefore strongly condemned, with natural deodorants advised instead. To replace needed fluids, drinking six to eight glasses of water daily, in addition to other liquids, is typically advised.

Occasional rash due to sweating and chafing may be difficult to avoid although frequent bathing and avoiding peak sun exposure may help. Cayce's soothing suggestion for skin irritations is a special kind of talcum powder containing tolu or Peruvian balsam and zinc stearate that has a gentle, drying effect:

> Should there continue to be the irritation of the skin, use some good powder—as Stearate of Zinc Powder—with Balsam. Use this for the rash that occurs on parts of the body.   69-6

Despite our best efforts to avoid them, insect bites and poison ivy are occasional environmental hazards. Palliative relief for both may be found in Cayce-recommended Ray's Ointment and Ray's Liquid, which contain ingredients such as sulfur, zinc oxide, pine tar, salicylic acid, phenol, and lanolin. Homeopathic Rhus-Tox is also sometimes advised for poison ivy symptoms.

When allergens such as pollen are present, probably the best general strategies are to avoid peak times of day, drink plenty of liquids, and keep one of Cayce's inhalant formulas on hand. Following a former A.R.E Clinic recommendation of five to seven daily drops of castor oil on the tongue can also be helpful. However, the most effective strategy of all is prevention. For this purpose the readings recommend ragweed itself brewed as tea or taken in tincture form:

> These will prevent, then, the recurrent conditions which have been and are a part of the experience of the body. This will enable the body to become immune because of the very action of this weed upon the digestive system, and the manner it will act with the assimilating body, too.   5347-1

Those who experience muscle soreness from exercising too much, too soon may appreciate a penetrating liniment consisting of olive oil, mineral oil, witch hazel, benzoin tincture, sassafras oil, and coal oil:

> It'll be necessary to shake this together, for it will tend to separate; but a small quantity massaged in the cerebro-spinal system will *take out* the inflammation or pain! 326-5

Other readings recommend a combination of equal parts olive oil and tincture of myrrh to benefit the muscles and superficial circulation. Typical instructions are to warm a small amount of oil before adding the myrrh.

The specter of skin damage caused by overexposure to the sun is ever-present during the summer months. However, it can be easily avoided by limiting direct exposure to those times of day when the rays are actually beneficial, such as early morning and late afternoon. Both are ideal times for walks, swims, yard work, and other outdoor activities that cannot take place in the shade.

To keep the skin lubricated and counter the drying effects of exposure to the elements, the readings suggest a variety of skin-nourishing formulas made from natural substances. When asked for a general skin care formula, Cayce's response was a specific combination of peanut oil, olive oil, lanolin, and rosewater with the comment:

> This will not only . . . give the body a good base for the stimulating of the superficial circulation; but will aid in keeping the body beautiful; that is, {free from} any blemish of any nature. 1968-7

Summer has paradoxically become a time of staying extra cool and extra busy while nature calls us to experience the heat and indeed the indolence that goes with it. Sometimes we just have to get out there and sweat!

Water Cures

Water is such an integral part of our makeup that therapeutic applications of it are many and varied, starting with a baby's first bath. Since we spend gestation floating in the primordial water of life, it's no wonder that humans usually regard water as soothing, cleansing, uplifting, energizing, healthy, and magical.

Hydrotherapy, defined by physiotherapist H.J. Reilly as "the science of the application of water in all its forms for healing and health," has been around for many thousands of years.[27] Sanskrit texts mentioned baths and remedies as early as 4000 BC. Water therapy was quite familiar to the ancient inhabitants of Tibet, Egypt, Crete, Babylon, Persia, and Greece before Rome got into the act. We have a long tradition of aqueous folk remedies to draw on!

The numerous Cayce readings on the subject use hydrotherapeutic methods as builders of health:

> . . . the care of the body in general—keeping plenty of water for the system, internal and external . . . will build the body to its normal resistance.   583-4

Many of these methods are outlined in detail in *The Edgar Cayce Handbook for Health Through Drugless Therapy*, which devotes two chapters to internal and external hydrotherapies.

The readings regard external hydrotherapy as an all purpose way of normalizing body functions by stimulating circulation and promoting elimination of toxins through the skin and lungs:

> For the hydrotherapy and massage are preventive as well as curative measures. For the cleansing of the system allows the body-forces themselves to function normally, and thus eliminate poisons, congestions and conditions that would become acute through the body.   257-254

The main external measures involve various types of baths. The examples given here can all be practiced with simple preparations. As in the above quote, baths were often to be followed with massage using oil.

---

[27]Harold J. Reilly and Ruth Hagy Brod, *The Edgar Cayce Handbook for Health Through Drugless Therapy* (New York: Macmillan Publishing Co., Inc., 1975), 204.

Hot baths of 101–104 degrees F (a thermometer is strongly advised) are an effective way to ease muscle aches and stiffness. After twenty to thirty minutes in the water, it's time to cover-up and rest for at least half an hour.

Warm baths of 90–101 degrees F are recommended to lower blood pressure, dilate blood vessels, and relax the nerves. A few drops of balsam or pine oil may be added for a relaxing effect. Again, it's important to rest or sleep afterwards for the full effect.

Cold baths are a way to enhance energy by stimulating the heart rate, increasing breathing, and revitalizing the nerves. Each short dip in 40–55 degree F water is preceded by a warm bath. A starting duration of one and a half minutes may be gradually increased to two or three.

Sitz baths are recommended in many readings and regarded by Reilly as "one of the most rewarding uses of water."[28] Cold sitz baths have been used to increase circulation, relieve congestion in the lower abdomen, counteract fatigue, promote elimination, indirectly relieve headaches, and even induce sleep. The idea is to cover one's back and shoulders with a towel and lower oneself into six to nine inches of tap temperature (60–65 degrees F) water with feet braced above the water level. After one minute's immersion (which can be increased over time), at least ten minutes of rest or sleep are advised. Since cold baths should always be taken when the body is warmed up, hot sitz baths can precede cold ones.

Shower baths, valued for their circulatory and tonic benefits, can take the place of tub baths if desired. In this method, warm water is run over the lower back while gradually increasing the heat for three to five minutes. Then cold is allowed to hit the warmed area (not the head at first!) for about forty seconds.

Epsom salts baths are considered highly therapeutic for stiff joints, muscle pain, arthritis, rheumatism, and many other conditions. For a standard tub bath, approximately five pounds of salts are required. The salt is dissolved in several inches of water at 101–102 degrees F and then more hot water is added, raising the temperature to 106 to 108 degrees

---

[28]Harold J. Reilly and Ruth Hagy Brod, *The Edgar Cayce Handbook for Health Through Drugless Therapy* (New York: Macmillan Publishing Co., Inc., 1975), 214.

F. With repetitions, a starting time of ten or twelve minutes can be gradually increased to twenty minutes. These baths are not advised in cases of high blood pressure or heart conditions.

Epsom salts hand and foot baths can bring relief to stiff, painful joints. The hands should be worked under the water and rubbed with peanut oil afterwards.

Fume baths, also known as cabinet sweats, are one of Cayce's favorite methods of promoting cleansing. This type of sweat is like a sauna with steam, which can carry a variety of therapeutic substances, such as benzoin tincture, lavender oil, eucalyptus oil, myrrh tincture, pine needle oil, witch hazel, tolu balsam, or wintergreen oil. If a steam cabinet is not available, probably the best method is to contain the steam produced by a vaporizer in the tub.

Internal hydrotherapy is another word for flushing, either of the digestive system by drinking water or of the large intestine through colonic irrigation. In the first method, Cayce's injunction is: "Well to drink *always plenty* of water, before meals and after meals . . . " (311-4) Six to eight glasses of good quality water daily are considered about right for health maintenance, and it's best to start early:

> Well, then, each morning upon first arising, to take a half to three-quarters of a glass of *warm* water; not so hot that it is objectionable, not so tepid that it makes for sickening but this will clarify the system of poisons.   311-4

In a colonic the large intestine is gradually flushed with several gallons of water to relieve accumulations on the intestinal walls and thereby normalize intestinal functions. Both colonics, which are performed by professionals, and enemas, which can be done at home, have a stimulating and corrective function:

> For, *every* one—everybody—should take an internal bath occasionally, as well as an external one. They would all be better off if they would!   440-2

The final form of water cure I will mention is more fun, freely avail-

able, and close. August is an ideal time for enjoying the cooling, energizing benefits of salt water immersion at the beach. After a dip, why
not try a sand pack, especially recommended for people living in or
visiting Virginia Beach because of the therapeutic gold content found in
the local sand. Simply allow yourself to be buried to the neck in a relaxing mound of hot, dry sand for ten minutes or more, and then jump
back in the ocean to rinse off. A real treat!

According to Reilly:

> Water, in its multitudinous uses, variations, and effects, is unpar-
> alleled as a therapeutic agent. It is as fluid in application as its
> own nature. It can relax, stimulate, relieve pain, heal, and purify
> the body internally and externally. It functions in a manner that
> cannot be duplicated by any other modality, with maximum
> stimulation of the body's own healing powers and a minimum of
> after-effects. Its very naturalness and flexibility make it possible
> to adapt this therapy to any degree of delicacy or strength of ap-
> plication dictated by the patient's condition. It is readily available
> (or was until we polluted it) and it is cheap.[29]

The "fountain of youth" is closer than we think.

More Precious than Gold

What is dearer to us in this world than our most valued metal—a
measure of wealth through history and throughout the world? One
obvious answer is our health. It gets interesting when something treasured for its sparkle turns out to have potential for putting some sparkle
back in us. No, we shouldn't start eating our jewelry, but the Edgar
Cayce readings propose some fascinating ways to experience the benefits of this precious mineral for ourselves.

Cayce's most common approach, when dealing with a perceived need
for gold in the body, is to utilize the principle of vibration. Using subtle

---

[29]Harold J. Reilly and Ruth Hagy Brod, *The Edgar Cayce Handbook for Health Through
Drugless Therapy* (New York: Macmillan Publishing Co., Inc., 1975), 207-8.

energy devices such as the Wet Cell and Radio–Active appliances is a truly brilliant way of transmitting the benefits of this (and other) minerals without the toxicity of internal dosage. Both of these devices can be attached by means of wires to glass jars containing mineral solutions, such as gold chloride in this case. Although the solution never comes in direct contact with the body, it apparently stimulates the system to produce the needed element on its own.

The readings have this to say regarding mineral solutions in general:

> We find that any of such solutions may be given to the body, as we have indicated, through this manner; causing the activity of same without it passing through the system itself, for it may be directed to various organs of the system that are in need of such elements—as to the glands in any portion of the system that receive impulse from the cerebrospinal system, or from the sympathetic or the vegetative system, or from any of the ganglia of the *lymph* or *emunctory* circulation that forms itself in portions of the body.
>
>   1800-25

The Physician's Reference Notebook by Dr. William McGarey and others contains quite a bit of commentary on the therapeutic use of the Wet Cell with gold in solution:

> The atomic effect of gold was said to be necessary for the glandular production of the hormone which maintained the proper structural condition and functioning of the nerves . . . The readings indicated that the vibration given from the gold in solution would be electrically transmitted into the body and have the glandular effect described above. Reading 1800-6 . . . suggested that the vibration did not act directly, but only enabled other elements (perhaps gold already in the body in an inactive form) to become active and have the desired effect.[30]

---

[30]William A. McGarey and Associated Physicians of the A.R.E. Clinic, *The Physician's Reference Notebook* (Virginia: A.R.E. Press, 1996), 268–69.

Used in this way, gold performs a central role in therapy, as its vibration can be harmlessly carried straight to the central nervous system. This capacity of gold to stimulate the nervous system was regarded by Cayce as a valuable element in numerous external treatments. Many doctors' commentaries found in *The Physician's Reference Notebook* make this point. Others try to make sense of the hazards of gold deficiency, concluding that it could cause a "glandular imbalance, in turn resulting in a hormonal deficiency or imbalance, disturbing proper functioning of the nerves."[31]

After all these remarks on the importance of administering gold by vibration, it may be surprising to find other forms of usage—in fact over two hundred of them! One type of short-term internal administration involving gold chloride and bromide or bicarbonate of soda is often to be followed by Violet Ray applications. The readings find this helpful in " . . . assisting the eliminations, aiding the system to function through the glands—where assimilation has been hindered, that causes tautness in the centers about nerve ends, where they join in the joints or sinews of the body." (120-2)

This only hints at some fascinating applications, and implications, for gold in the readings that those who are interested will have to research for themselves. Those who are familiar with phrases like "gold treatment" and "gold cure" are on the right track.

Finally, many local Virginia Beach residents and summer visitors to the A.R.E. have a firsthand familiarity with sand packs recommended at least in part for their gold content:

When there is the sand and sea bath, it is well that the body be covered with sand afterward—dry sand. Let the body be thoroughly wet in the sea water—this meaning with the bathing suit and the body thoroughly wet—and then immediately cover the body in *dry* sand, see? not wet.   849-33

The radiation from the gold and radium in the proportions that

---

[31]Ibid., 265.

you find in Virginia Beach . . . is the better for the conditions of the
body.   5237-1

That there is hidden value in coating ourselves with sand is something some of us have always suspected.

The Silver Solution

Hand-in-hand with gold, more often than not, comes silver—the precious metal we associate with the moon and intuitive wisdom just as
we link gold with the life-giving sun. A search of Cayce readings on the
subject yields just over five hundred documents, and a look at about
half of these documents reveals a surprising array of references ranging
from healing to financial advice.

The over seventy references to silver in healing vary as well, but
most have to do with correcting mineral deficiencies in the body in
some way. Apparently, elements essential to health are often lacking as
in reading 924-1 which notes a shortage of no less than nineteen minerals including silver. Diet and supplementation are only two ways of
providing these essential elements as the readings make so clear. Here is
where Cayce's subtle energy devices such as the Wet Cell and Radio-
Active Appliance come in.

Through the attachment of glass jars containing specific mineral solutions, both of these devices are evidently able to transmit the vibrations of these minerals to the system in a beneficial way. Speaking of
silver nitrate and gold chloride used together (typically alternated), reading 986-1 offers:

> Attached in these manners, the solutions carried to the body—
> through their activities through the vibratory forces of the electri-
> cal vibrations—would materially aid in establishing an equilibrium.
> For the centers in the system from which there arises these im-
> pulses would be *quickened* by such vibrations.

Other readings draw more distinction between the two elements,
referring to " . . . the Chloride of Gold, that will make for a change of

activity in the blood cellular force as to the creative energies—and the Nitrate of Silver, that will make for a change in the impulse in the nerve forces themselves." (1242–1)

In the appliance readings, silver and gold are usually found together due to their complementary nature:

> The Gold, which is carried into the system vibratorially through the Appliance, is to act upon the elements in the nerve system so as to renew the energies in same. The Silver is to enable the activity of the eliminating system to so eradicate the effects of the suppression of activity in the muscular and tendon forces as to allow same to be eliminated from the body.   1698-2

> These influences are found, then, in Gold and Silver in a form in which their vibrations may be accorded and assimilated to the living organism to give it greater strength, greater vitality . . .
>
> 887-4

> . . . given properly—silver and gold may almost lengthen life to its double, of its present endurance.   120-5

However, there are also some exceptions to this complementary practice. For instance, reading 1029–1 comments that:

> The principle or activative force in such attachments is that the Nitrate of Silver solution would act as a stimuli to the properties assimilated in the system, creating that necessary balance carried through the electronic energies of the body to and through the areas that have been affected and that become affected at times in the body at present.

Similarly, reading 1931–1 refers to "the stabilizing influence of silver," and one progress report states that case 1242 "finds the treatment with the Silver Nitrate solution very soothing—it puts him to sleep and gives him rest." Also readings in a number of cases regard silver as the metal of choice for the plates that are attached to the body with both appliances. Even one silver battery pole for the Wet Cell is occasionally advised.

Cayce's more miscellaneous references to silver are interesting in their own right. Fourteen individuals received counsel regarding mining ventures, hunts for buried treasure, or investments. Eleven were told that they had an affinity with silver from past lifetimes involving metal work, jewelry making, or commerce. Silver was also one of the colors to be used in constructing eleven aura charts (or life seals), which may be described as highly individual emblematic paintings designed to inspire and awaken soul qualities.

A few more references appear in the course of dream interpretations while others pertain to the silver cord described by the psychically gifted as a glowing kind of thread that keeps our earthly and soul bodies connected during a lifetime. For instance, reading 254-68 states that "the activity of the psychic forces operates in the material body, as we have outlined; along the pineal, the leyden and the cord—or silver cord." In this context, a person who is close to death, as in 226-2, is "about to sever the cord."

In yet another and final vein, both silver and gold appear in the course of spiritual counseling directed to close to forty individuals. In response to questions regarding financial support, wherewithal, and security, the readings typically advise strengthening spiritual foundations and trusting in God to provide—all in highly biblical terms. Reading 1151-24 enjoins: "Remember—Whose is the silver and the gold?" The vast majority begin with: "The silver and the gold is mine," saith the Lord," and then go on to paraphrase parts of Psalm 50 as a reminder of the Creator's infinite abundance.

Part of the "silver solution" is, therefore, always a note of gratitude for its shining presence in our lives.

The Remarkable RAP

The Radio-Active Appliance, a.k.a. Impedance Device, Radial Appliance, and more recently Radiac, is perhaps the most unusual and promising of the many and various therapeutic "gadgets" found in the Edgar Cayce readings. In fact, as a subtle energy device, it may still be ahead of its time, making it especially topical today.

Since there's nothing nuclear about this appliance, many have wondered why Cayce consistently regarded it as radioactive. The answer may be as simple as early definitions of radio, or "wireless," or perhaps the readings are comparing the vibration produced between the battery and its user to the resonance of a radio wave.

In any case, the other names came later. The term Impedance Device, found in some readings' reports, is an electrical one probably having to do with Edgar Evans Cayce's description in a 1965 report of the battery as "simply a capacitor and a resistor in parallel."[32] The term Radial, which occasionally appears in the readings, refers to the radiation of emanations or rays. Radiac is a more recent contraction of radio and active. "RAP" is a personal favorite.

There's really nothing electrical about this appliance in the conventional sense. It's actually quite futuristic in that it doesn't plug into the wall but instead is charged by direct sunlight and then activated by ice water just before use. It doesn't generate a measurable electrical current either, although it's designed to affect the body's energy field, which has often been described as electrical in nature.

At any rate, the Cayce source is enthusiastic enough about this unremarkable looking device to recommend its use in well over four hundred readings, which sometimes include instructions for making it. A typical comment is: "This is beneficial to *anyone, properly* used!" (1884-2) Certain logistical considerations and a strong emphasis on holding a devotional attitude during use to avoid harmful boomerang effects are then often added.

Cayce's own descriptions of how and why the RAP affects the flow of body energies have huge amounts of information to offer. Here are some examples:

For, as the vibrations are controlled through the activity of the Radio-Active Appliance, this takes energies in portions of the

[32]Edgar Evans Cayce, *Two Electrical Appliances Described in the Edgar Cayce Readings* (Virginia: A.R.E. Press, 1972), 3.

body, builds up and discharges body electrical energies that re-
vivify portions of the body where there is a lack of energies stored.
                                                                    3105-1

The effect of this application is to keep the circulatory system
balanced between the sympathetic and cerebrospinal, stimulating
the glands along the whole system where there is the cross activity of the vibrations of the body; creating a more normal balance,
giving strength and enabling the body to rest better, thus enabling
better mental and physical activities of the body.   478-3

While the Radio-Active Appliance is non-electrical in its reaction, it
does produce the *proper* coordination in the upper and lower portion of the circulation; thus is conducive to rest and ease.   515-1

The low electrical vibratory forces . . . {are} the basis of life. The
application of such vibrations to the body when it is fagged in
mind, in physical endurance, will stimulate the necessary influences for the body to return to the abilities within self to carry on
. . .   444-2

The Radio-Active Appliance is good for *anyone,* and especially
for those that tire or need an equalizing of the circulation; which is
necessary for anyone that uses the brain a great deal—or that is
inactive on the feet as much as is sufficient to keep the proper
circulation.   826-3

. . . coordinating of the physical body with the mental body creates that which is commonly known as memory. An assistance to
this will be found in the use of the Radio-Active Appliance, which
is well for everyone . . . But if we will allow a perfect physical body
to coordinate with the activities of the influences about it, it *creates* a memory.   416-9

One effect of a better coordinated body is evidently an improved
ability to deeply relax during sleep:

. . . And then *whenever* there are the periods of overtiredness, overanxiety, the desire on the part of the body for real rest, use same—the Appliance.   1022-1

And this will be . . . a type of appliance for bringing rest to the weary . . . to those who have been under great periods of stress and strain; to those who seek to find an equalizing influence that will assist them in producing a coordination in their physical and mental beings with the spiritual affluence and effect of its activity of spirituality upon the body-physical.   1800-28

Restlessness . . . and irritation will disappear.   1472-2

Perhaps it is this calming effect that makes the RAP effective as a meditation aid, especially during the times when it is actually in use:

And use that period, when the Appliance is attached, for meditation; when the body would meditate upon its purposes in the earth, its thanks and praise to the living God; its desires to be the channel for a blessing, for a helpful experience, for the knowledge of God in the life and experience of others.   2800-1

Use the period when the Radio-Active Appliance is attached as a period not of conversation but rather of contemplation and meditation, as periods in which the body will review its own experiences in the earth, its relationships and that the body is planning to do with its life in relationships to others, and as to the reasons for the body being in the material experience in the present; and what it intends to do with the opportunities for being an expression of its ideals in this sojourn.   4030-1

. . . these {days} will be found to be, if it may be so termed, the "lucky" days, or the periods when there is a closer association with Creative Forces about the body.   1179-1

In short, it sounds like this little battery is just what the doctor or–

dered for keeping body and soul together. This makes it an ideal "youthing" aid:

> And if the body were to use for its own physical body the Radio-Active Appliance . . . it may keep its body in almost *perfect* accord for many—many—many—many—*many* days.   823-1

That Revivifying Violet Ray

Those who are familiar with the body's seven major energy centers may already be picturing some sort of third eye emanation. Sounds like fun, but in this case the reference is to yet another intriguing electrical device widely recommended in the Edgar Cayce readings.

The Violet Ray, so named because of its crackling purplish electrical discharge, is mentioned well over eight hundred times. An invention of the famous Nicola Tesla, this device harnesses high voltage, low amperage static electricity in a clear glass applicator with a handheld base. Today it is commonly referred to as a high frequency device and should not be confused with ultraviolet lights or sun lamps.

Although it is now familiar primarily to beauty parlors, the Violet Ray was used for a wide variety of medical conditions with applicators to match in the first few decades of the last century. The readings subscribe to some of these uses and in other cases probably invent new ones.

In the readings the static electricity produced by the Violet Ray is regarded as beneficially stimulating to both the superficial circulation and the nerves. In the process other helpful effects can be achieved. For the circulatory system the results are described as both toning and balancing:

> This would be to create a balance of circulation through the superficial portion of the body, causing a bettering of the conditions.
> 436-4

> This will make for the abilities of the body to rest better. It will tend to make for strengthening of the body, by the toning of the circulation—as combined with the adjustments that are taken. 1611-2

The effect of the Violet Ray on the nervous system is described as calming and invigorating at the same time:

> If this is taken just before retiring it should aid in the ability to rest, and quieting the nerves.   540-12

> This treatment is to so charge the centers . . . as to make for . . . better coordination *between* the sympathetic and cerebro-spinal nervous system. It would produce stimuli to the *ganglia* in the . . . coordinating centers.   259-7

> . . . apply to the body the correct vibrations that will give the incentives to the nerve centers to become rejuvenated again . . .
>   269-1

Coordinating Violet Ray treatments with spinal adjustments or massages over the same areas can be especially beneficial:

> Thus not only would the distresses in those particular portions be relieved, but the impulse for the circulation through the head and neck and to the optic forces and to all portions of the face would be such as to *improve* the functioning of the organs; bringing a nearer normal condition.   679-2

> The osteopathic adjustments, and especially the heat from the high vibrations of the violet ray in the manner indicated, will aid.
>   1540-3

> This may be taken at the same periods when the preventative measures are taken for the strengthening of the muscular forces in the lower portion of the body, by the gentle massage . . .
>   772-3

The Violet Ray's stimulating effects were often employed in cases where the body had not been moving well and its "batteries" were low:

And the activities of the violet ray are only to make for the electrical rejuvenation of nerve energies that have been depleted through
the inactivity of the whole system of the body.   676-1

This will give the "pick up" or the stimulation that is needed for
what might be called the recharging of the centers along the cerebrospinal system, so that there is better coordination between the
ganglia of the cerebrospinal and the sympathetic nerve system.
                                                             1196-17

. . . To do this will prevent the central nervous system batteries
from running down . . . It'll pick the body up!   2528-4

Even the body's elimination functions can be aided at these times:

Apply across the abdomen very thoroughly, that we may awaken
the functioning of the liver, spleen and those portions in the digestive tract.   979-3

. . . the vibrations of the . . . violet ray . . . will aid in *equalizing*
with the rest of that applied the general circulation and nerve distribution . . . With these corrections, and especially with the vibrations of the Violet Ray applied in the manner given, these will
create more activity through the eliminating *systems*, and *especially* through the alimentary canal.   5640-1

Perhaps the best-known use of this appliance is in the care of the
hair and scalp:

. . . using the comb of such a hand violet ray machine through the
hair and head, will make for such stimulation as to make more
growth of the hair and also a better growth of the hair.   1120-2

The Violet Ray is also a standard treatment in cases where the mind
has been overcome by negative influences:

These treatments will tend to make for the raising of the vibrations of the body, disassociating the effects of repressions in the system, producing better coordination throughout.   1572-1

Because the Violet Ray is an electrical appliance, the usual precautions are indicated along with several more from the readings. Users are warned to avoid all medicinal substances, including Atomidine, on the same days. This warning extends to alcohol in any form, including Cayce's own inhalants. As one reading puts it:

Abstain from *any* intoxicating drinks of *any* kind! This means even beer, too! Too much of these, with the electrical forces (if they are to be taken), will be *detrimental* to the better conditions of the body.
    Electricity and alcohol don't work together! It burns tissue, and is not good for *anybody!*   323-1

Other readings warn against spinal adjustments, X-rays and Kriya yoga exercises on treatment days. Still others advise keeping applications short, especially in the beginning:

Do not overstrain, but keep the violet ray—and not more than the minute and a half.   1861-11

With these precautions in mind, perhaps commencing treatments after the holidays would be best! Times of new beginnings are just right for pausing to recharge. And if using a Violet Ray for this purpose: "Apply it in such a manner as to expect and to obtain the revivifying of the body-forces themselves." (3060-1)

Feeling Good about Massage

Though it's not unusual to find Cayce treatment modalities with hundreds of recommendations, massage just about tops the list—with over twenty-five hundred! There are many excellent reasons why being rubbed the right way is vital to health.

Probably number one is the fact that massage works its magic externally without messing with sensitive body chemistry. In other words, it's minimally intrusive and at the same time capable of far-reaching internal benefits—an unbeatable combination.

Another notable feature is that massage promotes absorption of helpful elements from the formulas and oils used on the skin. Although a fully clothed chair massage is always better than no massage at all, the readings contend that using natural oils such as peanut oil, olive oil, and lanolin will magnify therapeutic potential.

Then there's the remarkable healing power of touch itself. Cayce's repeated suggestion of nightly back rubs shows more concern with consistency and therapeutic intent than with the availability of trained professionals doing evening outcalls. The main requirement for performing this task is someone who cares.

Many exciting findings on this topic have come out of the University of Miami, School of Medicine's Touch Research Institute. For instance, massage in the workplace has been used to induce relaxation and heighten alertness at the same time—while no doubt increasing job satisfaction! Healthy touch has also been a helpful element in weight loss programs as well as in treatment of eating disorders such as anorexia.

Perhaps most exciting is the use of massage, with oil in particular, to help babies grow and thrive. In one study, regular, gentle stroking sessions helped premature infants to gain weight so they could leave the hospital as soon as possible.[33] Further research published in 1997 suggested that massage improves an infant's ability to process information.[34] A third study published in 1996 concluded that massaging babies with oils (as opposed to without) enhances parasympathetic activity, producing a powerfully calming effect.[35]

Since receiving bodywork is much more fun than reading about it,

---

[33] F.A. Scafidi et al., "Massage Stimulates Growth in Preterm Infants: A Replication," *Infant Behavior and Development* (April–June 1990): 167–88.

[34] M. Cigales et al., "Massage Enhances Recovery from Habituation in Normal Infants," *Infant Behavior and Development* (January 1997): 29–34.

[35] T. Field et al., "Massage with Oil Has More Positive Effects on Normal Infants," *Pre and Perinatal Psychology Journal* (Winter 1996): 75–80.

we will now proceed to some experiential suggestions. A good start is to schedule a professional massage at least once a month if only to help the body remember how it feels to completely unwind for an extended length of time. You can, then, begin to extend the intervals of deep relaxation arising from these appointments by exchanging back (substitute head, neck, shoulder, foot) rubs with family members or friends. Even children usually love to give as well as receive massage, and their hands are surprisingly strong and caring. Couples and friends are apt to discover a nurturing new form of communication. If awkwardness is an obstacle, remember that there's only one cure for inexperience. The two exercises that follow are a good start.

The Top Three Cayce Strokes

Anyone can learn the basics of a Cayce-Reilly back massage. Have the receiver lie face down on a table, bed, mat, or soft carpet with the entire spine bared. Positioning yourself at the head, lubricate clean hands with the Cayce formula or oil (try peanut or olive) of your choice. Begin by sliding the hands slowly and firmly down the back from the shoulders to the hips, running your thumbs along either side of the spine. Then drag your hands back up using equal speed and pressure. This is your beginning and ending stroke. It cannot be repeated too many times.

After at least six repetitions, position yourself on one side and prepare to knead the entire *opposite* side of the back. Beginning with the shoulder area, move slowly downward, alternately pushing one hand away while pulling the other toward you in a "rolling and kneading" motion. When you reach the hips, reverse your direction toward the shoulders, repeating the entire circuit at least three times. Include the sides as much as possible, using the thumbs to apply extra pressure to any areas that seem tight. Reposition on the opposite side and repeat.

Remaining on one side, use the middle two fingers of either hand to make a series of small circles along the spine, beginning at the base and moving gradually upward. When you reach the top, circle slowly back down. Each circle should press up and outward. Switch hands and circle up and down the other side. Repeat as often as desired.

Reposition yourself at the head to end the massage with long, slow strokes.

The "Couch Potato"

This is an ideal introduction for any duo lacking in successful massage experience. No disrobing is required except for the removal of shoes and socks. Clean feet are obviously a plus.

In this simple and rewarding exchange, one person sits on a couch or comfortable chair with the other seated in front and below, on the floor or a cushion. The person in the upper position can now easily rub or knead a partner's shoulders, upper back, neck, and head without tiring very quickly. Meanwhile, the person below can begin to massage the other's feet, bringing one foot at a time into the lap. Anything goes, from stroking, pressing, and friction to stretches and bends. The key is to keep up a running dialogue on what feels good and what does not so that each partner can learn to please.

After five or ten minutes or more, switch positions. Caution: you may become so drowsy that you lose interest in the TV!

Both of these simple massage practices are guaranteed to move anyone out of the head and into the body—where consciousness belongs at the end of a demanding day. Who knew that experiencing one of the oldest and most effective forms of preventive medicine could feel so good?

Just Pack It! Part I

We often need reminding of the importance of packs, which in physiotherapy lingo refers to masses of wet, sticky, or otherwise gooey substances applied to various parts of one's anatomy for the purpose of therapy. This may only sound like fun to those with a highly developed inner child, but it's never too late to wake up and smell the Glyco. The truth is that packs—and their close relatives poultices and stupes—are deeply embedded in our folk traditions as well as the Edgar Cayce readings. The basic ingredients are as close as a well-stocked medicine cabinet—or the kitchen.

Castor oil with around six hundred recommendations is Cayce's top, and possibly, gooiest pack material. Usually regarded as too strong for internal use, this castor bean extract has both soothing and penetrating properties when placed in contact with the skin. Abdominal applications—the usual kind—are broadly intended to induce relaxation and promote normal processes of elimination, though their effects can be much further reaching. In the readings, the oil is regarded as a softening agent:

> . . . the application of those things that may *soften* this area that is distressed—or the packs of castor oil. Apply at least three to four thicknesses of flannel wrung out of castor oil as hot as may be handled with the hands or received by the body; across that portion of the abdomen on the right side and across to the left, you see. We find these will materially aid.   261-12

Castor oil's amazing capacity to penetrate below the skin's surface is enhanced by heat, usually by way of an electric pad or a bag of hot salt (more later). In cases where extra heat is contraindicated, such as pregnancy or inflammation, one option is to simply apply the pack at body temperature.

A type of mini pack often combining castor oil with baking soda or camphor is advised in about fifty readings. A piece of gauze with tape is perfect for small trouble spots on the skin.

Mutton tallow is a key ingredient in several hundred formulas intended to draw the circulation to areas that need warming. The tallow (or suet), which is derived from sheep, is a uniquely penetrating lubricant that in this case serves as a carrier for the absorption of other substances. The most typical combination is equal portions of mutton tallow, spirits of turpentine, and spirits of camphor, sometimes with the addition of benzoin tincture or sassafras oil.

The usual practice is to heat the formula and rub it into any areas that need the stimulation, which can include the chest, neck, throat, ears, upper back, kidney area, feet, and lower limbs. These areas are, then, kept warm using towels or a source of heat:

Apply about head, ears and neck an equal combination of Mutton Tallow, Turpentine and Camphor. Keep it . . . as warm as possible without burning, until there is the draining of same—either from nasal passages, throat or ears.   2036-6

Stimulate those areas through the chest and over the lower portion of the lungs, so that the congestions there, the lymph flow through these, the tendencies for the soft tissue in the head and face, may be cleansed; by using the hot applications *(with a hot salt pack)* . . . For this combination makes for a loosening of the congestions through these areas . . .   1045-2

An **Epsom salts pack** is a type of wet application (stupe) advised in another several hundred readings to promote relaxation and reduce discomfort. This pack is made by dissolving Epsom salts in hot water to make a saturated solution, meaning no more can be absorbed. Cloths are then dipped in the solution, wrung out, and applied as warm as possible to affected areas. Hot towels are then applied to help retain the heat.

This is a localized alternative to the often–recommended Epsom salts baths. Pack locations vary widely with the areas of discomfort involved. These include arms, legs, upper spine, lower spine, abdomen, kidneys, and joints:

This will make for the relaxing quickly . . .   298-2

This will relieve the pain and produce activities that will make for an *easing* of the disorders in the system.   243-12

This . . . will assist in relaxing the system sufficiently that the circulation—both in the nerve and blood supply—may have effect upon the organs of the system that are disturbed, producing that condition wherein the applications—that may be used daily—may effect the absorption and elimination of the disturbing forces . . .
                                    357-1

Dry salt packs are highly recommended in a couple of hundred readings as a steady, deeply penetrating source of heat. While heat is often considered therapeutic in itself, the right kind of salt (iodized, sea, raw) can be a healing factor in its own right. Hot salt is often used here to promote relaxation while enhancing the effect of other types of packs, including Glyco–Thymoline and those already mentioned. As with Epsom salts packs, application sites are determined on an individual basis.

In this type of pack, the salt is encased in a cloth bag of the desired size and heated in a low temperature oven (microwaving might be ideal). Cayce explains:

> Over this pack use salt heat—not just a bag of heated salt, but sew the salt into a container—quilted, as it were. Heat this in the oven and apply over the Glyco-Thymoline pack, instead of using an electric pad. Preferably use iodized salt; not so hot as to burn, but let the body lie upon or over the Pack.   987-5

Wow! We've only covered four kinds of packs—not nearly enough. But, be of good cheer, more packs will come to light in the next chapter, and we'll even venture into the kitchen!

Just Pack It! Part II

As promised, we now continue our exploration of the drippy, goopy, wild, and wonderful world of therapeutic packs.

Vinegar and salt packs are another type of stupe; in this case it consists of regular salt (from a natural source) dissolved in hot apple cider vinegar. In more than one hundred cases these are advised over areas such as the knees, hips, lower spine, elbows, hands, and shoulders to provide a deeply penetrating source of wet heat. Apparently the vinegar and salt combination carries special benefits:

> {We will} bring to this portion of the system a renewed activity . . . by application of properties as would be found in pure apple vinegar and salt (hot) . . .   33-1

> Make this rather thick, see, and not so wet that it becomes runny

but damp sufficient that the body is absorbing the chloride from
same . . .   303-16

Mullein stupes are advised in probably less than fifty cases to relax
the muscles and have a strengthening effect. Sites and frequency of
application vary widely. Some readings recommend drinking mullein
tea during the same course of treatment. Here are some Cayce instructions:

> For those places on the limbs and the body where there are swell-
> ings, we would prepare Mullein Stupes. But do not have same too
> hot or too cold; just a little above body temperature. Prepare same
> in hot water and then put leaves on a very thin cloth, like dressing
> cloth. Then put a heavier cloth over same and apply to the body.
>   304-44

> Not give these except when the body tired, that the system calls
> *for resuscitating* forces, see?   409-10

Grape poultices appear in close to forty readings as a method of
supplying strengthening properties to the body. These packs are always
to be applied over the abdomen without heat and changed each time
they become warm until relief is obtained:

> Put a poultice of grapes, cool—grapes of any character, prefer-
> ably Concord . . . we want those with seed for it's the tartaric acid
> that we are giving that we want the reaction from. Crush same,
> place between thin cloths over the abdomen, extending up to the
> lower end of the stomach . . .   304-34

> This is to assist—not only by the absorption—in supplying nour-
> ishment to the circulatory forces through the portion, but in giving
> strength to the body; as well as keeping the bodily forces in ac-
> cord in the circulatory force.   308-5

Glyco-Thymoline packs are a preferred approach in about thirty readings. Sites of application, which vary with the individual, include the throat, chest, lower back, knees, feet, abdomen, and hips. However, the usual favorites are the neck and the sinus areas on the face:

> On the throat apply three to four thicknesses of cotton cloth saturated with Glyco-Thymoline, full strength, normal temperature, not heat applied.   1112-9

> We would use the Glyco-Thymoline packs over the nasal passages, or sinus passages. Saturate three to four thicknesses of cotton cloth, or gauze, in warm Glyco-Thymoline, and apply over the passages, allowing such a pack to remain on for fifteen to twenty minutes at the time—and keep up until the passages are clear. Apply such packs whenever there is any distress . . .
>   2794-2

These packs are easily done with a cotton washcloth folded to the appropriate size and shape. In cases where heat is indicated, a dry salt pack is preferable.

Onion poultices, a classic folk remedy for severe congestion, can be found in about twenty readings. In this treatment raw onions are ground up presumably in order to make them juicy (a food processor would work well), and then lightly heated, sometimes mixing in a little corn meal. This mixture is then spread on the chest, covered with gauze, and replaced every four hours or so, until breathing is easier. Here are Cayce's instructions:

> We would prepare an onion poultice; grind the onions and put in a sack, . . . and apply over the throat, the chest, and those portions in the upper and even to the lower part—where there is the heaviness.   710-2

> On the frontal portion we would put an Onion Poultice, for activity to the circulation through the breast, the chest and the lungs, see?
>   303-40

Potato poultices are found in twenty readings as a kind of drawing agent for cleansing and relief of eye irritations. In this treatment raw white potatoes (again, use organic) are scraped to form a mush. This soothing substance is then applied directly to closed eyelids. Although old (perhaps meaning the baking variety) potatoes were always specified, this does not mean they should have "eyes" or be in the sprouting stage. In Cayce's words:

> For the local applications to the eyes (because of irritation of the lids), we would use scraped Irish potato; using a good antiseptic to bathe same off when the compact of the potato is removed.
>
> 340-46

> If there is the continuing of inflammation, we would use of evenings the scraped Irish potato (old potatoes, not new ones) on gauze applied to the eyeballs themselves, or sockets, see? Let this remain on for a half to three quarters of an hour.   2086-1

Last but not least is the delightful messiness of **mud packs** used for their drawing, cleansing, and stimulating properties over the face and elsewhere. At least fourteen readings recommend the application of various types of clays for health and pleasure. On an occasional basis, these natural astringents are a refreshing way to give the face and neck a healthy glow:

> The *best* is with that of the *mud* bath, or those applications that will *cleanse* same—in the *muds*, see?   255-10

> But once a month, for the very pleasure of it, we would have the mud pack.   1968-7

This is what it really comes down to for those who give packs a chance—a luxurious feeling of pure spa-like enjoyment. The body feels warmed and coddled, nurtured and cleansed, and usually ready for a nice healing rest. Don't be concerned if the tune running through your head becomes a parody of a Michael Jackson song: Just pack it, pack it . . .

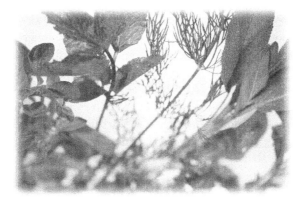

Common Concerns and Disorders

Throat Coat, Be Gone!

S o, you haven't quite "come down" with anything yet, but your body's feeling stressed and your throat's a little scratchy and you're avoiding the high notes at choir practice. Or, you've dripped and sneezed your way through a cold or the flu, and you're basically okay now except for this wicked little throat tickle that's playing havoc with your sleep. Both scenarios are prime opportunities to slow down, relax in a steaming bath, down plenty of fluids, and head to the Cayce medicine chest for some old-fashioned remedies.

A nice, strong gargle is a great place to start. If you've never felt the power of Atomidine to unload mucus from the throat, this must be experienced to be believed. (Caution: do not use this full strength. Follow dilution instructions on the label.) Atomidine is a versatile product with over six hundred recommendations that harnesses the properties of iodine to promote expectoration from mucous membranes. If traces of the solution remain in the mouth after gargling, additional benefits may occur. Versatile Atomidine " . . . may be used for the dental, the hygiene, and the internal . . . " (358-1)

A milder but in many ways equally attractive alternative is Glyco-Thymoline, a pleasant–tasting liquid recommended as a mouthwash, gargle, skin soother, and mucous membrane alkalizer in over eight hundred readings. This latter feature is important because of categorical assertions by the readings that alkalizing the system is to the cold virus what immersion in the lava of Mount Doom was to Tolkien's ring of power. Originally promoted by its manufacturers as a *treatment for mucosity* (when labels could make such claims), this unique formula has a truly restorative effect on congested throats. If swallowing a few drops is unavoidable, that's okay too because "The Glyco-thymoline acts as an intestinal antiseptic of an alkaline nature . . . " (3104-1)

If annoying throat tickle is a persistent problem but you prefer to avoid suppressants, a soothing blend of herbal extracts may be just the thing. For instance, the tonic combination of wild cherry bark, horehound, rhubarb, wild ginger, honey, and alcohol found in reading 243-29 is intended to act as a "cough medicine, an expectorant, and for a healing through the whole system . . . It will allay the cough, *heal* those disturbing forces through the bronchi and larynx, and make for better conditions through the eliminations."

Use of a grain alcohol-based inhalant formula is another extremely effective way to promote expectoration. In solutions of this type recommended in well over two hundred cases, substances such as tolu balsam, eucalyptus, benzoin, turpentine, and creosote act as a form of respiratory aromatherapy. Fumes produced when the liquid is shaken are typically inhaled by means of a breathing tube. Though inhalation may cause more coughing at first, the end result is often spectacular relief. The readings speak of a " . . . reaction from the gases for the throat, bronchials, lungs, that not only heal but that prevent accumulations from poor circulation through the muco-membranes of throat, nasal, bronchi . . . " (421-8) Ah, the sweet inspiration of relief!

Smoothing Scars

Everyone has "battle scars" marking the spots where the skin's surface has been breached and a repair made. Much like the mending of holes in a sweater, the small repairs barely show, but big ones can end up looking messy. The Cayce material on this topic points out that the smooth healing of injured tissue goes far deeper than simple cosmetics because the scar becomes a kind of roadblock to normal circulation in that area.

An example is a reading for a fifteen-year-old boy that recommended daily massage of his scarred left limb to "reduce the most of this." When asked whether removing the scar would lead to any health improvements, Cayce replied:

> Any scar tissue detracts from the general physical health of a body, for it requires changing in the circulation continually. Not that the massage would injure the body, but would make for better physical health generally.   487-15

With excessive scarring regarded as a health issue, it's easy to understand why so many readings focus on helping the skin to heal as smoothly as possible. Usually this is to be done through massage in which various substances are rubbed in and around affected areas. The central ingredient in these liniments is camphorated olive oil used either alone or in combination with other substances such as peanut oil and lanolin:

> Q. What should be done to dissolve scar on forehead?
> A. The use of camphorated oil twice each day is the best application for removing . . . scar tissue on any portion of the body.
> 1566-4

Camphor, or *Cinnamomum camphora* (also sometimes known as laurel camphor or camphor laurel), is a very interesting botanical. The camphor tree is a close relative of the cinnamon tree and is native to eastern Asia. Camphor crystals and camphor oil are made from the glossy dark green leaves, roots, and wood chips of the tree. In addition to its purely aromatic uses, camphor is a common ingredient in massage formulations, lip salves, and inhalants. The oil is used therapeutically to ease bruising, inflammation, and joint pain.

The Cayce readings subscribe to most of these uses and add a few more where camphor is recommended for various external purposes in almost seven hundred readings. Several advise using camphorated oil made with olive oil rather than the more typical cottonseed. Here is a fascinating explanation:

> . . . olive oil—properly prepared (hence pure olive oil should always be used)—is one of the most effective agents for stimulating muscular activity, or mucus-membrane activity, that may be applied to a body . . . The Camphorated oil is merely the same basic force . . . to which has been added properties of Camphor in more or less its raw or original state than the spirits of same. Such activity in the epidermis is not only to produce soothing to affected areas but to stimulate the circulation in such effectual ways and manners as to combine with the other properties in bringing what will be determined, in the course of two to two and a half years, a new skin!   440-3

In other words, camphorated olive oil and Cayce's other scar formulas stimulate and soothe the skin at the same time. While they increase the circulation both in and around the healing areas, the possible irritation of still tender skin is allayed.

At least one reading—this one for a three-year-old girl—suggests that camphor preparations were already being used for this purpose in Cayce's day:

> Q. Will continued use of Camphorice gradually eliminate scar on arm (resulting from severe burn 2 years ago)?
> A. Camphorice, or better—as we find—Camphorated Oil. Or make your own Camphorated Oil; that is, by taking the regular Camphorated Oil and adding to it; in these proportions:
>
> Camphorated Oil .... 2 ounces,
> Lanolin, dissolved .... ½ teaspoon,
> Peanut Oil .... 1 ounce.
>
> This combination will quickly remove this tendency of the scar— or scar tissue.   2015-10

Whether camphorated oil is used plain (on older scars only) or diluted as in the above formula, using it on scarred areas once or twice daily should be enough to make a visible difference. It may even be possible " . . . to prevent or remove scars, as the tissue heals." (2015–6)

As with many other Cayce treatments, dogged application over what may seem like an extremely long period of time is said to be the key to success:

Massage this each day for three to six months and we would reduce most of this.   487-15

. . . remember the whole surface may be entirely changed if this is done persistently and consistently.   440-3

Correcting Constipation

The start of a new year is an ideal time to take a really close look at what continues to keep us going—or not. Even a glance at the remarkable variety of laxative products on drug store shelves tells us that "irregularity" is, indeed, a major concern. Due to factors inherent in the modern lifestyle, such as refined foods, inadequate water, lack of exercise, and stress, many of us are simply not evacuating wastes in the proper manner. As a result, constipation—defined as inadequate, difficult, or infrequent evacuation of the bowels—is distressingly, and dangerously, common.

Even in today's climate of growing health awareness, many who suffer from constipation are largely unaware of the causes and the risks. However, those mildly unpleasant symptoms, such as gas, bloating, queasiness, and a lack of get–up–and–go, are apt to become more serious unless the disorder is corrected at its source. Moreover, Cayce and some prominent health authorities agree that constipation can lead to more human ills than any other single condition.

In other words, proper elimination along with its corollary—the effective assimilation of nutrients from foods—is central to health. The readings even go so far as to state that a person with these two functions working perfectly can renew the body indefinitely:

There should be a warning to *all* bodies with respect as to such conditions; for . . . would the assimilations and the eliminations . . . be kept nearer *normal* in the human family, the days might be extended to whatever period as was so desired; for the system is builded by the assimilations of that it takes within, and is able to bring resuscitation so long as the eliminations do not hinder.

                                                                        311-4

Descriptions in the readings of how constipation originates are quite consistent. A key feature of early development is hyperacidity—due to emotional tension and/or poor diet—in the region of the stomach and duodenum. The excess acid impairs both lymphatic and liver functions, creating a deficiency in enzyme production, which, in turn, affects both assimilation and elimination. At this point, even familiar foods, which would normally be digested with ease, suddenly begin to disagree, causing indigestion. As a result:

Intestinal indigestion produces packs *[impaction]*, and this in turn produces the condition in the colon known as constipation. Constipation in turn produces re-absorption of toxins. Toxins produce taxation to the nervous system. The nervous system produces taxation to the brain and sympathetic system. Hence we have that tired, dull, achy feeling, and the tendency to feel every bodily ailment that may come to the body, see? We have a complete cycle in these physical conditions.   550-1

Other common contributions to this escalating cycle are misalignments in various areas of the spine and a consistently acidic diet. If the sources of constipation are not addressed, toxicity increases, liver function is impaired, the kidneys are under stress, and skin disturbances as well as halitosis may result. Headaches and infections are common as conditions worsen, and the specter of colon cancer—rare in Cayce's day— looms on the horizon.

Cayce's instructions for correcting this condition vary with its severity and the nature of related ailments. In chronic situations, intestinal cleansing is a typical first step. Gentle laxatives of plant and mineral origin are usually to be alternated when continued over any length of time. Specific products mentioned include Innerclean, Castoria, Zilatone, olive oil, and a blend of sulfur, cream of tartar, and Rochelle salt. At the same time, antacids and stomach soothers, such as limewater and charcoal tablets, are advised to improve digestion. Colon cleansing by means of colonics or enemas is another frequent suggestion.

Spinal adjustments are often needed, as well, to relax nerve centers in the lower spine and relieve pressures interfering with proper elimination. Treatments would typically take place two or three times a week for several weeks.

Another prescription both for overcoming constipation and preventing a recurrence is a highly alkaline diet. The consumption of up to 80% of vegetables and fruits along with whole grains, legumes, the lighter proteins, and six to eight glasses of water daily (between meals) will virtually guarantee intestinal health. An occasional fast, such as the well-known three-day apple diet, is strongly advised.

The importance of constructive attitudes and emotions should not be underestimated. Anxiety and the holding of grudges may be the worst culprits as they can " . . . bring about barriers to proper reactions throughout the system; whether as related to the circulatory forces or the assimilations or eliminations of the body." (816-8)

Once the intestines are working more normally—and often!—vigorous exercise is one of the best forms of preventive medicine. A daily walk, a swim, a bike ride, a stretching routine, or an aerobic workout have a host of benefits that keeps our systems working more regularly in every way.

Natural Help for Hearts under Pressure

February's focus on the heart reminds us to lovingly watch for potential issues before they get out of hand. This is especially true physically of conditions that can lead to heart disease, such as hypertension.

Abnormally high arterial blood pressure is an extremely common condition that can severely compromise one's health. Millions die prematurely each year as a result of this destructive disease. Possible causes for hypertension include nervous tension, kidney disease, localized narrowing of the aorta, and arteriosclerosis, or the hardening of the arteries in the elderly. However, most cases are categorized as essential hypertension, meaning there is no known cause, although heredity and excessive salt intake are considered possible factors.

With notable exceptions, the general rule in hypertension is that the higher the pressure, the greater the cardiovascular damage. A chronic increase in arterial pressure will lead to enlargement of the heart, followed eventually by congestive failure. A decline in blood supply to the heart is also a common result. If the pressure is regarded as high enough to seriously damage the heart, drugs come into play. These medications are typically continued for life, and there can be undesirable side effects.

Approximately one hundred Cayce readings address the problem of hypertension and related issues. Some of these individuals were already experiencing the serious consequences of heart disease while others were told that their condition was not yet organic, meaning that the heart itself had not been permanently damaged. Described essentially as a circulatory system imbalance, the elevated pressure in these cases is regarded as the end result of a combination of factors, which vary somewhat with each individual.

One common focus of concern is the alignment of vertebrae in the lower thoracic (6th to 9th) segments of the spine located near the heart. Misalignments due to injury or internal stress typically lead to nervous system imbalances and "laxness" of nerve centers disturbing the flow of circulation to the digestive system and/or heart.

Another common root cause is found in problems of a gastrointestinal nature. Difficulties with assimilation, elimination, or both will eventually impair the functioning of the liver and lead to absorption of toxins by the system. The result is an excessive volume of blood and a "plethora" or overabundance in the flow to the heart.

The readings also sometimes focus on the role of attitudes and emotions in disorders of this type. Anxiety, nervous tension, and repressed anger are among the contributing factors cited.

All of these readings propose helpful measures to reduce the elevated pressure and bring, at least, some relief. Basically, they focus on the delicate matter of equalizing the circulation and correcting underlying problems while avoiding further strain on the heart.

Readings in many cases give instructions for adjusting vertebrae in the thoracic area as well as in other parts of the spine. The use of massage or heat is also sometimes indicated to thoroughly relax the affected areas.

A light diet is frequently advised until the pressure has been reduced. Typical instructions are to focus on vegetables and lean proteins while avoiding fats, pork, and most starches and sugars. A need for greater water intake is highlighted in quite a few cases as is going extremely easy on meat and not eating at all when excited or overtired.

Internal prescriptions vary widely. Many readings advise a variety of herbal preparations with tonic and cleansing ingredients.

In cases of toxicity a primary treatment is irrigation of the large intestine to gently reduce the pressure in the colon. For those with nervous system imbalance, the Wet Cell is sometimes the treatment of choice. In the more serious cases, getting plenty of rest is strongly recommended until the heart is able to function with less strain. Light exercise is suggested where appropriate.

Since follow-up reports in the cases examined are few, it seems probable that many either did not follow their readings or were too ill to recover fully. An exception was Mr. 4345, who responded: "I wish to report that I am feeling much better, having followed your advice over a period of about six months. I find my physical condition greatly improved and my blood pressure very materially reduced."

Lower pressure would be a wonderful valentine indeed!

Arresting Arthritis

If health police existed, they would say that when one's gait starts to stiffen, muscles to ache, and joints to enlarge, the culprit is probably arthritis, a pervasive degenerative disorder that plagues tens of millions in the US alone. Although the term refers primarily to inflammation of the joints, it also serves as an umbrella for a number of other related malfunctions that affect the musculoskeletal system. Of the hundred-plus different types of arthritic disease, the two most common are osteoarthritis, caused mostly by wear and tear on the large weight-bearing joints, and the more disabling rheumatoid arthritis, which may affect many of the smaller joints as well.

The many discourses in the readings on this topic can be distilled into several main areas of focus. Those that follow can be applied to various types of arthritic disease.

According to Cayce, most cases of arthritis can be traced to a functional imbalance between the body's organs of assimilation and elimination with chronic deficiencies in nutrient intake and waste management affecting each other in a debilitating kind of progression. There are also chemical changes involving glandular imbalance and circulatory abnormalities in a system that is literally being poisoned by toxins originating in the gastrointestinal area. With the body in emergency mode, proper rebuilding of cells in the joints and ligaments is sacrificed.

In reversing this process, the first order of business endorsed by Cayce is, therefore, to promote internal cleansing through diet and other treatments. A typical arthritis diet in the readings consists of easily digested vegetables, fruits, whole grains, and light proteins. A decrease in meat and carbohydrates is often advised, or meat may be completely eliminated for a period of time with the exception of beef juice. Foods with a laxative effect, such as in the "mummy food" combination, are common. Sugar, refined grains, fried foods, carbonated drinks, beer, hard liquor, and white potatoes (except for the skins) are to be avoided with few or no exceptions.

Additional aids to detoxification, especially in the form of castor oil packs, enemas, and colonics, are often recommended. Epsom salts baths and cabinet sweats, which promote elimination through the pores of the skin, are preferred in the most sensitive cases.

Poor or impaired circulation is often regarded as a contributing factor in arthritis. Circulatory deficiencies can easily contribute to gastrointestinal sluggishness leading to an aggravation of symptoms.

Cayce's primary solution to this problem is gentle massage, especially in cases where little else can be tolerated. This is usually to follow an Epsom salts or steam bath, which relaxes the body and promotes the absorption of oil. Cayce's favorite for this purpose is peanut oil. A combination of equal parts of heated olive oil and a tincture of myrrh is also often favored. Other massage formula ingredients suggested include lanolin, pine needle oil, sassafras oil, witch hazel, wintergreen oil, and cedarwood oil.

When it can be tolerated, the readings also advise spinal manipulation to improve the circulation, relax the muscles, relieve pain, and alleviate pressure on nerve impulses to all parts of the body. In the view of the readings, there is no other form of mechanical therapy so closely in accord with the natural attempts of the body to heal from within. Also recommended, where appropriate, is light to moderate exercise.

Glandular imbalance is found to be a factor in development of many cases of arthritis. The endocrine glands, which secrete hormones capable of activating specific organs, play a vital role in maintaining the body's chemical balance. When this balance is chronically upset by intestinal problems, the resulting toxins can lead to arthritis symptoms.

Glandular stimulation is, therefore, often indicated to help dissolve deposits in the joints so they can be gradually drained and eliminated. Treatments such as Epsom salts baths and massage are employed for this purpose.

Another important cause of arthritis, which begins with its ruinous effect on digestion, is negative attitudes and emotions. The readings put it this way:

As indicated for most people and it is very well here: don't get mad and don't cuss a body out mentally or in voice. This brings more poisons than may be created by even taking foods that aren't good.   470-37

Constructive attitudes in action may be regarded as both treatments in their own right and supplemental to others. One way to creatively apply the concept of "mind is the builder" is to literally reinforce an expectation of health by always visualizing treatments as beneficial.

Several other Cayce arthritis treatments deserve mention but are more individualized. They include hot Epsom salts packs over painful areas, various forms of electrotherapy (Wet Cell, Radio–Active appliance, Violet Ray, Ultra Violet Light), and tiny internal doses of gold and soda.

How does one come up with a personalized arthritis treatment? A possible approach is to find a reading that seems to "match" one's case. Another is simply to focus on the basics of correcting the diet, adding elimination aids, scheduling regular massage, promoting glandular stimulation, and adopting healthy attitudes. The clear message is that arthritis symptoms may be arrested and, in time, dissolved—as surely as an well-deserved chance for parole.

Unseating Piles

Hemorrhoids or "piles" are among those "unmentionable" complaints in which a little shared information can bring a huge amount of relief. In fact, initial results can be quite speedy although the root causes naturally take more time to address.

These irritating sac-like formations in the lower portion of the rectum and tissues around the anus are basically composed of enlarged and varicose veins. The primary symptoms are itching, bleeding, and some level of discomfort. Symptoms may worsen over time to a point where surgery is required.

The extremely common nature of this complaint does not mean it should be considered normal. According to the hundred-plus Cayce readings on the subject, hemorrhoids are but one sign of an entire body out of balance. Dr. William McGarey described four typical factors in their development: hyperacidity, constipation, emotional stress, and disturbed hepatic circulation linked with autonomic nervous system imbalances. Here's what happens next:

> When eliminations are decreased, the assimilation of foodstuffs into the body is lessened, the lack of nutrient elements creates glandular deficiencies, anxieties, and often an increased acidity. The lymph is suppressed, irritations arise; incoordinations develop between parts of the nervous system and the deep and superficial circulation; the hepatic circulation and the balance between the eliminatory channels are all upset.[36]

---

[36]William A. McGarey, MD and Associated Physicians of the A.R.E. Clinic, *The Physician's Reference Notebook* (Virginia: A.R.E. Press, 1996), 173.

To put this chain of events in Cayce's words:

> Hence an excess of acidity has at times caused the folds of the
> sphincter centers, and the lower portion of the alimentary canal,
> to become involved in the disturbance because of the very lack of
> the lymph and the elimination through the proper channels of the
> excess drosses in the system.   257-199

The first order of business in these cases is always symptomatic relief.
For this purpose Cayce's many recommendations begin with a specially
formulated ointment known by the rather quaint name of Tim. This
combination of butterfat, benzoin tincture, powdered tobacco,
Atomidine, and sometimes other ingredients is to be applied to affected
areas as often as needed:

> The directions would be to apply as an ointment to affected por-
> tions once or twice each day. Rest as much as possible *after* appli-
> cation, with the feet elevated *above* the head. It'll cure it!
>   1800-20

A drugstore product known as Pazo is sometimes suggested as an
alternative to Tim. Often advised in addition to either ointment was a
kind of healing enema solution composed of glycerin, carbolic acid,
and heavy mineral oil:

> Thus the character of enema indicated is not only to act as a heal-
> ing influence and to prevent the folds reforming, but is to allay the
> disturbance and prevent the tissue that has broken from becom-
> ing scar tissue and again causing disturbance.   404-8

To help reduce discomfort and prevent future outbreaks, the readings recommend the famous "piles exercise" of rising on the toes with
the arms above the head and then bending forward, still on tiptoe, until
the hands have touched the floor (or the air above it, as the case may
be):

This done several times each day, very slowly, will gradually lift the sphincter muscle and thus remedy the hemorrhoid condition.

3678-1

In acute situations ice packs are always helpful as are castor oil packs in the experience of the former A.R.E. Clinic.

With relief underway, it's time to systematically correct underlying causes and instill healthier habits. This means alkalizing the diet (more fruits and veggies, less junk); aligning the spine (with the help of an osteopath or chiropractor); correcting constipation (using the methods of one's choice); applying hot packs across the low back while discomfort persists (with Epsom salts solutions or castor oil packs); exercising regularly (especially walking), and building constructive attitudes (through prayer, gratitude, ideals, and inspirational reading).

Incidentally, there are two stories in circulation on the origin of the name Tim. One is that it is based on the initials of some of the ingredients: tobacco, iodine and menthol. The other, from Gladys Davis, is as follows:

The name Tim was given in the readings themselves after our good friend, Mr. [195], whose nickname was Tim, prepared the formula indicated in his own reading and, getting good results, continued to make it in those early days for others who had it advised in their readings.[37]

Since the formula comes in a very small jar, it could even be called "Tiny Tim" with the appropriate Dickensian blessing applied during use!

The Joy of Holistic Childbearing

Nowhere is health more vitally important—on the part of both progenitors involved—than in the creation of new life. Because we are far more than just physical beings, this statement applies on a variety of

---

[37]An Edgar Cayce Home Medicine Guide (Virginia: A.R.E. Press, 1986), 107.

levels, which are aptly explored in Cayce's approximately seventy readings on the subject. Consistently emphasized is the sense of wonder and privilege that engaging in this supreme creative act is meant to evoke:

> For no greater office is there for an entity to fill than to be a channel through which a soul may find the way of experience into the material plane.   480-30

In this vein, women who had either conceived or were preparing to do so were repeatedly counseled about the dynamics of spiritual laws such as soul attraction, soul choice, and karmic responsibility:

> Here is something that each and every mother should know. The manner in which the attitude is kept has much to do with the character of the soul that would choose to enter through those channels at that particular period.   2803-6

Holding an attitude of spiritual expectancy during the entire experience is regarded as especially desirable:

> Keep the attitudes for the mother in the manner in which there may be known that those who bring a soul into activity in the material world have those privileges, opportunities, for the giving of an expression . . . that with the development of that soul . . . may not only make for joy and peace and harmony in the experience of that soul but be an added condition for manifestations of God's love to the sons of men.   575-1

Because like attracts like, those who consistently spiritualize their attitudes through prayer, meditation, ideals, and so forth will naturally attract souls who are spiritually oriented themselves and who will enrich the lives of others:

> For, as you each—now—are responsible for that channel through which a soul may manifest in materiality; then in love, in faith, in

hope, in prayer, *prepare* that channel that *that* soul—that may be drawn through those activities that are in preparation—may be as one that may be a blessing to not only those upon whom the body is dependent, but through that it may give of itself in and as a channel of hope, of blessings, to others.   934-3

According to Cayce, the attitudes held by both parents not only determine which soul will be attracted but are directly reflected in the personality and temperament of the expected child. The following advice is typical:

Keep in the attitude of creative forces. Keep happy. Do not let anxiety of any nature disturb. For it will have much to do with the nature or character of the individual dependent upon the body.
       23-16

Some readings, utilizing the often-cited principle of "mind is the builder," suggest practicing a form of creative visualization during pregnancy to influence developing patterns:

Keep happy, and keep that expectancy of that character and disposition that is desired in the offspring; knowing and realizing in self—as should be in the companionship—that this is being a channel for the manifestation of God's love in the earth. 2635-2

Other readings comment that interests and activities pursued by the mother to be are extremely influential and that even gender can be affected by a strong enough parental desire. This may be especially pertinent during the second trimester, which is regarded as critical developmentally because of all the marked changes that occur.

All of these high-flying considerations must, of course, be grounded in top quality physical care to optimize the health of both mother and child. Super nutrition is the largest building block in this scenario. The readings typically advise a balanced, highly alkaline selection of body and blood building foods, such as fruit, vegetables, milk, eggs, whole grains, seafood, and the lighter meats, such as poultry and liver. These foods are intended to strengthen the mother's resistance while building her baby's blood, bones, teeth, skin, muscles, brain cells, and other body tissues. The following guidelines are typical:

> Keep plenty of those things that are body and blood building, and that are not fattening—but that produce the greater quantities of the blood supply—the Vitamin B-1, as in cereals and all yellow foods. In the latter portion of the period, take plenty of milk. But now have plenty of fresh vegetables—these will tend to keep bettered conditions for kidneys and for body eliminations; fruits and vegetables, and especially those that carry the vitamins B-1.
>
> 2336-2

Although the readings often recommend certain vitamins and minerals, including A, B, D, calcium, iodine, iron, magnesium, phosphorus, and silicon, dietary sources of these nutrients are usually what they have in mind. Many prescriptions can be quite specific as in advice to ". . . eat a raw carrot once in a while if you want good eyes for yourself and your baby!" (1504-4) Supplements such as Calcios, cod liver oil tablets, B complex, and wheat germ oil are clearly food based as well.

Pregnancy is a time when the condition of the organs of elimination must be carefully monitored. Drinking plenty of pure water is advised as needed to keep the kidneys clear. Certain types of liquids, such as sodas, alcohol, and coffee, are usually to be avoided especially during the first trimester. In the second and third trimesters, precautions against straining the kidneys are coupled with recommendation of mild diuretics, such as watermelon, watermelon seed tea, diluted Coca Cola syrup, and water.

For bowels in need of stimulation, only the gentlest measures are advised. These usually take the form of enemas, colonics, and extremely mild laxatives such as Milk of Magnesia and Fletcher's Castoria. All other types of medications, including sedatives, are to be avoided.

Spinal manipulation once or twice a month is viewed as an outstanding way to enhance circulation, strengthen spinal and abdominal muscles, promote general relaxation, and correct specific imbalances. One reading accurately predicted that regular adjustments during pregnancy would result in real health improvement.

Recommendations of massage, which has many of the same benefits, are mostly of a general-purpose variety. Substances to be rubbed into the skin include olive oil, myrrh tincture, peanut oil, and cocoa butter. Backrubs are best taken at home when preparing to rest and do not have to be given by professionals.

Keeping a healthy balance between exercise and rest is especially critical during pregnancy. Walking is repeatedly recommended for its strengthening and toning effect on the lower body as well as the benefits of exposure to fresh air and moderate sunlight. Other types of exercise occasionally advocated include the head and neck exercise, stretching and bending from the waist, hip rotations, squatting, swimming, and dancing. Most are to be done regularly but in moderation.

The need for sufficient rest receives equal emphasis with cautions against overexertion of any kind. Activities to be avoided include straining, pushing, pulling, climbing, running up and down stairs, heavy lifting, and too much standing on the feet. Regular rest periods are also strongly advised.

If the Edgar Cayce readings on healthy childbearing were to be distilled into one thought, it might be that, just as with a recipe, we get out of it exactly what we put in with the element of surprise as an extra "special spice." It is our intentions that determine what goes into the mix and how we experience the result. A personalized affirmation articulating one's intention to become " . . . the more perfect channel for the manifesting of thy love to the children of men" (1749-1) is an ideal place to start.

Sleeping WELL!

There are few things in life so frustrating as being unable to fall asleep or stay zonked for very long when every instinct is yelling that deep relaxation is exactly what is needed. (Only those clearly of alien origin who have never had this problem will fail to sigh affirmatively here.) Worse yet is the spiraling insomniac cycle that can result when one bad night leads to enough anxiety and discomfort to provoke another.

Since the ability to rest well is such a vital key to health, the first imperative is to find a way to break the pattern of dysfunction with at least one sound, restorative night. Then it's time to take a hard look at the personal habits that support or detract from getting a good night's sleep. In many cases, one or two "no-brainer" resolutions, such as avoiding stimulants after a certain time or going to bed when one first feels sleepy, will work like magic. In others, it may be necessary to ferret out some deeper health issues or bow to sensitivity in this area by developing one's "bag of tricks." With the possibilities limited only by imagination, here are some places to start.

Diet and Supplements

Both muscles and nerves need a broad array of nutrients for daily energy and restful nights. The B complex vitamins and the minerals calcium and magnesium are vital to healthy nervous system function, and these minerals also play a role in proper muscle contraction and tone. Both omega-3 fatty acids and lecithin support the nervous system as well. A diet high in fresh, unrefined foods such as vegetables, fruit, whole grains, and light proteins such as eggs, oily fish, and dairy will provide these nutrients in abundance. However, extra nutrients may be called for in times of stress.

To make the most of their relaxing effect, take calcium and magnesium at night in a combined form easily found on health food store shelves. Specific Cayce-recommended calcium sources include Calcios, made from pulverized chicken bones, and limewater, a calcium hydroxide solution. For almost immediate yawns, try time-honored warm milk and honey. Cayce's preferred and most flavorful solution for bolstering the B's is B complex and iron in a liquid form.

Many herbs and other naturally derived substances make helpful relaxation aids. Members of the mint family (chamomile, peppermint, spearmint, catnip) as well as passion flower (especially advised by Cayce) and valerian are easily found in delicious tea blends as well as in tincture or capsule form. Melatonin, a serotonin derivative that's secreted by the pineal gland, is widely used to promote both relaxation and anti-aging agendas. Since the hormone regulates our biological clock and declines drastically with age, it's reasonable to expect that supplementation would improve both quantity and quality of sleep.

Exercise

Lack of exercise during the day is a proven recipe for restlessness at night. And, although exercising a few times a week does have proven benefits, it takes a daily routine to have a nightly affect. Any kind of workout stimulates the circulation to deliver nutrients, eliminate waste products, circulate lymph, tone the muscles, increase oxygen intake, enhance metabolism, and calm the nerves.

The readings mention many types of exercise, with walking the consistent favorite. Also often advised are a morning constitutional of upper body stretches, bends, and rotations and an evening cool down focusing on the lower extremities. Coupling evening stretches with some deep, slow, breaths can be truly yawn producing.

Massage

Much of our daily tension ends up as muscular in nature, regardless of how it originates. Massage is, therefore, one of the most direct pathways to short- and longer-term relief. It even has the added bonus of making up for a certain amount of lost sleep while it primes the body for more. Professional bodywork may be technically the most therapeutic, but it's hard to get at bedtime, which is undoubtedly one reason why Cayce often suggested relaxing rubs from family members. If said member balks at this request, why not offer to trade, say on alternate nights? If or when a hands-on rub is simply not feasible, chair massage pads and long-handled massagers can be extremely soothing.

Castor Oil Packs

This one may seem far-fetched until one tries it. There's something about having a warm, relaxed belly that can send a person straight into dreamland. There are actually several readings that suggest the packs for this purpose, and the improvement in sleep patterns from a single application can be truly remarkable.

Describing the sleeplessness as a type of "nerve tension," the readings typically advise at least one series of abdominal packs with heat taken for three consecutive evenings a week. The usual duration is at least an hour when ready to retire though it's fine to fall asleep with a pack in place and the heating pad off. Simply remove the pack and any excess oil on the next waking cycle. These packs are said by Cayce to have so many health benefits that deep relaxation can seem like a kind of bonus.

Water Immersion

Because of its calming, soothing nature, bathing is a pleasant way to slow our thoughts and reconnect with our bodies after a hectic day. Tub baths and swims are more effective than showers for this purpose. A few drops of an essential oil such as lavender or rose can extend the restful properties in creative ways. Bathing is, of course, an ideal prelude to a massage.

Reading

As a final sleep aid, consider this very article. Your eyelids should be getting nice and heavy right about now. And while you're in this receptive state, here's a posthypnotic suggestion: When you wake up, you'll have some wonderfully relaxing gift ideas for Valentine's Day. Sometimes a sweetie's soft smiling snores are the best reward of all.

Healing Gout from the Inside Out!

Many are all too familiar with gout—a condition where uric acid, one of the end products of protein metabolism, builds up in the blood. The arthritic attacks and joint inflammation, especially of feet and hands, can be truly excruciating. Despite the familiar cartoon stereotype of inflamed big toes, the excess acid may crystallize to form deposits almost anywhere in the body. Sudden attacks alternating with pain-free intervals are common, but symptoms may become chronic if not checked.

The typical victim of gout is a portly (this used to mean "well off") gentleman past the age of forty-five who habitually overeats and underexercises. An affliction known as "poor man's gout" is attributed to a combination of hard work, exposure, poor diet, and overindulgence in alcohol. Women are affected too, but in fewer numbers.

The Edgar Cayce readings do not mention gout by name but contain many references to uricacidemia, a condition with similar symptoms. The Uricacidemia Circulating File contains information given to only one man and eight women, all over the age of forty-five. Evidently most of these recipients did not consult Cayce until their condition had become acute and they were very uncomfortable. Affected areas mentioned include the heels, ankles, feet, knees, head, and side. Swelling, hives, food allergies, muscle aches, puffy eyes, and joint pain were common associated symptoms.

Uric acid deposits are viewed by the readings as resulting from long-standing imbalances coupled with a progressive deterioration of health. An acidic diet, viral infections, and congestion all produce relatively mild symptoms at first until the alimentary canal and colon literally become overloaded causing indigestion, poor assimilation, and inadequate elimination. Another often cited factor is spinal misalignments affecting the coccyx, lumbar axis, and sciatic nerves and thereby impeding normal circulation to the legs and feet.

The end result in every case is a severe strain on the body's waste disposal system impairing liver, kidney, bladder, spleen, and gall duct functions. Uric acids are not eliminated as usual and begin backing up into the blood stream instead, resulting in toxicity and circulatory imbalances with feelings of heaviness, sluggishness, and fatigue. Crystallization of these acidic deposits would lead to irritation, tenderness, and swelling, sometimes with incapacitating results.

Cayce's first advice to those afflicted with this distressing condition was to quickly correct its causes before what he described as functional disturbances became permanent. The good news is that, with persistent effort, the disorder can be reversed.

As might be expected, dietary changes are a central key to recovery. Avoiding pork, beef, meat fats, and fried food is an absolute must. Moderation is counseled with starches and sweets, although whole grains and honey are okay. The main recommendation is that one meal each day be a raw vegetable salad of lettuce, carrots, tomatoes, peppers, celery, and so forth. (Note: Be sure to also include celery seeds, according to renowned herbalist James Duke.[38] They're easily found on grocery store spice racks.) The salad can be accompanied by an oil dressing and perhaps some whole grain crackers or toast. Fruit, nuts, soup, and occasional seafood are also desirable.

Another important recommendation is spinal manipulation and/or massage. Usually a series of adjustments with special attention to the lower spine is required. Massage suggestions, which vary widely, include special attention over the liver and kidney areas.

Attention to all systems of elimination is no less important. Many were instructed to receive at least one high enema or colonic to relieve the pressures in the colon. Various types of laxatives and diuretics are found in almost every case. Several readings advise at least one three- to five-day series of abdominal castor oil packs, concluding each series with up to two tablespoons of olive oil internally. Hydrotherapy routines including fume baths and Epsom salts baths are sometimes suggested as well.

These readings propose some very specific treatment sequences, and how closely they were followed is not known. However, great improvement was reported in three cases.

Gout is clearly an extremely painful condition that anyone would want to avoid. If Cayce is correct, our best chance may lie in hitting the salad bar, avoiding heavy proteins, and developing a taste for celery soup. It's pretty good, actually.

Well-Soothed Soles

Our feet are what keep us up and running through life, and we already know how healthy it is to keep moving. It, therefore, be-hoofs us (pun intended) to treat our hard working pedal pushers with the tenderness and understanding they deserve. Luckily, the readings abound

---

[38]James A. Duke, *The Green Pharmacy* (New York: St. Martin's Paperbacks, 1997), 272.

in heeling advice that will aid us in putting our best foot forward.

This article is based on a survey of about two hundred readings yielding seventy or so references to the step-by-step care of our lower extremities. Two major themes run throughout this body of advice. The first is that the shape of the feet can reflect that of the body as a whole so that treatments are often indirect. The second is that applications to the feet and lower legs can influence that of the body as a whole, so treatments are designed accordingly.

The first theme is illustrated by Cayce's comments on most of the foot afflictions one can imagine including pain, irritation, arch problems, calluses, bunions, athlete's foot, muscle tightness, strains, dryness, stiffness, sore spots, and blisters. All of these ailments are, at least in part, considered symptomatic of poor circulation, which is in turn often due to "pressures" on the blood vessels and nerves serving the feet and lower legs.

For instance, case 457's large toe joint pain was attributed to a lack of circulation throughout the extremities. A person who asked about foot irritation and change in the shape of the nails was told: "It is the *contraction* of the nerve and muscular forces in the limbs making for the variation in the activities." (69-3)

Sometime later, Cayce added: "For, as has been indicated, when the circulation is slowed, the extremities are the areas that obtain the least of the proper impulse for the removal of used energies." *(69-5)*

In this same vein, a series of readings for case 243 linked pains in the toes with poor circulation through the lower limbs due to varicosity and later continuing pain in one foot to the effect of toxins in the system. Strain to the bursas of the feet experienced by case 400 was attributed to an injury to the lower back and hip.

In another case a condition resembling athlete's foot is attributed to: "The inclinations for the activities upon the feet to make for greater pressures in the axis of the lower lumbar area." (412-10) In fact, the readings regard spinal misalignment as a common factor in this ailment asserting that: " . . . this is almost *always* the condition where there is what is termed as Athlete's Foot or where the locomotaries are disturbed. That is, an impingement." (477-1)

The Cayce perspective on the origin of foot afflictions is even better illustrated by his treatments. In the case (above) of the irritated right foot, spinal manipulation was advised: "With the relief of the pressure on those portions of system that so easily affect the circulation from the lumbar area throughout the whole portion, we will find that these conditions will be relieved and improved." (69-3)

Later readings added massage of the limbs and feet along with advice regarding shoe inserts for proper arch support.

General massage, with special focus on the heel and ball of the foot, is another treatment of choice where injury is involved. This can be preceded by special types of stretches as in one of the conditions resembling athlete's foot:

> Standing flat upon the feet, gently rise upon the toes; do this for some six to eight to ten to fifteen times, gently; at the same time raising the arms gently with same during this lower portion of the activities. This will make for the proper circulation through these portions of the body.   412-10

This particular reading advises massaging with equal parts olive oil and tincture of myrrh, made by first heating a small amount of oil and then adding the myrrh:

> Massage all the body will absorb of this through the toes, across the instep and *thoroughly* into the soles of the feet. This will not only act as a local application for help but will strengthen the limbs.   412-10

Spinal manipulation and massage, both sole-soothing specifics, are especially helpful for weakened arches. An individual who asked about raising the arches was told: "The general applications with the leg and foot adjustments, in the general treatment, should correct these." (299-4)

Of course, the right shoes are also important: "Don't wear them {heels} too low, and we will find that those conditions that have been produced in the middle bursa of the foot will be better supported." (264-23)

Each type of foot problem naturally requires the right type of topical application to boost circulation. In the stronger formulations, ingredients such as Russian White Oil (a heavy mineral oil), witch hazel, grain alcohol, and sassafras oil are typical. Regarding this particular mixture, Cayce notes: "This would be good for anyone that stands on the feet much, or whose feet pain, or ankle or knees or tendons." (555-5) Similar formulas are sometimes given in cases of athlete's foot as are proprietary products such as Ray's Ointment and Ray's Liquid.

Different types of applications can be found in cases of localized irritation caused by calluses and bunions. One of these is a now extinct cream known as Dog-On-Foot, containing salicylic, benzoic, and thymic acids. In response to a request for a good callus treatment, one reading found that either Dog-On-Foot, an unknown product known as Foot Ease, or baking soda dampened with spirits of camphor would do the job, but that the last combination " . . . will make for the removal of same with less certainty of it coming back again." (270-34)

Another reading describes this same formula as " . . . good for anyone having callous places or any attendant growths on feet, for it will remove them entirely!" (276-4) Softening of hardened areas can also be accomplished with castor oil and baking soda or sometimes with castor oil alone.

When looking at foot treatments intended to aid the body as a whole, massage makes a lot of sense. Stimulating the circulation in the feet and legs induces general relaxation and indirectly boosts blood flow throughout the body. This is also the case with heating the feet in conditions such as colds and congestion. One Cayce favorite is bathing both feet in an old-fashioned mustard bath made by stirring a teaspoon of the powdered spice into a couple of gallons of piping hot water and then " . . . rubbing the feet and limbs to the knees or above the knees thoroughly when the feet are put into the water. See? This would stimulate the circulation to the lower extremities and take it away from the head, until the eliminations have cleansed the system sufficient that there may be started the proper circulation." (558-4)

Another common treatment for congestion is to massage a combination of mutton tallow, spirits of camphor, and spirits of turpentine into the feet and then keep them extra warm. This might or might not follow a stimulating mustard soak.

A final method of boosting the superficial circulation is by means of the Violet Ray, which can be applied directly to the lower limbs or in a manner resembling the Radio–Active Appliance. In the latter case, the applicator is alternately held in each hand and placed in contact with each foot in a specific rotation, such as right hand, left foot, left hand, and right foot. A more balanced circulation to the extremities is apparently the effect desired.

It should be evident by now that Cayce's foot care measures are really pretty modest. One doesn't have to be especially well heeled or need someone else to foot the bill. A reflexology treatment may be all that's required to keep us toeing the line. So, take a stand for sole satisfaction, try a little hip–hop, and never admit de-feet!

Sweetening the Stomach

It's moving on toward bedtime, and your stomach just can't seem to settle. Or worse yet, there's a child whose stomach can't seem to settle, and you are called upon to DO SOMETHING.

Well, there are a number of over–the–counter drugstore products you could reach for, but a lot more choices are available to the holistically inclined. Cayce's digestive helpers are gentle, soothing, and sometimes even taste good.

Probably the simplest thing to start with is a nice relaxing cup of herbal tea. Chamomile is a mild–tasting digestive stimulant and stomach soother commonly found in bedtime blends. The readings recommend the tea by itself and in combination with others used for similar purposes, such as saffron and elm:

This will act with the gastric juices of the stomach to supply those necessary forces that will be needed in the digestive system to prevent this taxation . . .   2176-1

{It will help} . . . to create more of a muco-membrane in the stomach and intestinal system, see? . . .   2884-3

Camomile tea and Saffron tea altered from time to time, a little of

these in place of water at times, will settle the stomach and make
for the releasing of the irritations.   712-1

This, as we find, will reduce inflammation throughout the mesenteric system.   4204-1

Chamomile tea is easily prepared by pouring hot water over a pinch
of the herb in a teacup. Some readings, however, advise making a more
concentrated solution that can then be added to cool water as needed.

Saffron is another tea alternative recommended in about two hundred and fifty readings for its beneficial effects on digestion, assimilation, elimination, the stomach lining, and the skin. The following
comments are typical:

The Saffron will assimilate and coordinate with the gastric juices
of the *digestive* system, in such a way and manner as to eliminate
that character of poisons that saps the vitality of the muco-membranes *of* the digestive and intestinal system.   4510-1

These properties as a tonic or stimulant in the assimilating system
would produce and keep, with the digestive forces, the proper reactions as to prevent recurrence of disturbing conditions . . .
                                                                        556-16

It stimulates better strength through the activities of the lymph
and emunctory circulation in the alimentary canal.   257-215

The saffron once or twice each day, that the irritation may be kept
down and *preventing* any re-occurrence.   348-5

Again, this tea is made by steeping a pinch or so of the herb in a
teacup of hot water. Then it can be cooled before drinking if desired.

Elm water, suggested in about one hundred and seventy readings,
apparently has similar soothing, stomach coating effects. For many,
Cayce advised:

Well that occasionally those properties in the elm . . . be given as an easing for the conditions in the stomach proper.   2190-1

If this is belched, then reduce the quality but keep on taking.
                                                                                261-22

Should this become offensive, in that it produces belching from non-activity through the system, discontinue and take Yellow Saffron water, or tea, see?   356-1

Many readings advise alternating elm and saffron for best results:

There should be no water taken unless carrying elm bark or Yellow Saffron tea. While these may be in small quantities, the effect of these upon the gastric flow throughout the stomach, throughout the activity of the organs of the system, will so stimulate the walls of the organs themselves as to bring *healing* to those portions that are distressed.   745-1

Elm water is prepared by stirring a pinch of powdered slippery elm bark into a glass of cool water a few minutes before drinking. It has a mild slightly sweet flavor.

Limewater and cinnamon water are digestive and stomach settling aids found separately and together (often with other ingredients added) in several hundred readings. Rather than a citrus product, limewater is a saturated solution of slaked lime (calcium hydroxide). As an alkalizing liquid and a source of calcium, it appears in readings for babies, children, and pregnant women.

Cinnamon is a sweetly fragrant bark that is often used as a flavoring agent in foods. Cinnamon water is made by dispersing a single drop of the essential oil in eight ounces of water.

Lime and cinnamon water are always combined just before use by adding just a teaspoonful of each (perhaps less for children) to half a glass of water, milk, or juice. The readings have this to say about their effect on the system:

We will find that the pains, or the bloating, will be eased most by

equal parts of lime water and cinnamon water . . . This may be
given whenever there is any distending. This will ease . . . 193-2

On such a voyage (if a voyage taken), use those of equal parts of
cinnamon water and lime water as an alternative for the settling of
the stomach and digestive system.   142-5

Take a little lime water and cinnamon water, equal parts, if there is
the nausea of morning.   711-4

Coca–Cola syrup, though advised in a much smaller number of cases,
is an easy remedy for stomach distress that was a medicine chest staple
at the time when the readings took place. Small amounts of this syrup
(a tablespoon or two) diluted in water evidently have a settling and
diuretic effect that is extremely beneficial for some bodies:

Coca-Cola or the like, if it is prepared from the syrup and using
plain water (not carbonated water), will not be harmful; in fact, it
would be helpful for the kidneys and for the purifying of the blood
flow.   2766-1

Charcoal tablets are an old–fashioned option for indigestion, belching, and gas. In these cases the charcoal acts as an adsorbent, meaning
that it adheres to troublesome molecules of gas and liquid until they
can be safely eliminated:

Too, we find that the Charcoal Tablets would be well for this body,
as they absorb the poisons and the tendencies for accumulations
where there is the discharge of eliminations from used energies to
the alimentary canal.   1100-13

The brand usually recommended at the time was made by Dr. Kellogg
of the Battle Creek Sanitarium. However, these tablets made with willow
charcoal and honey are no longer available. Other brands are possible
substitutes.
    Finally, pepsin is a digestive enzyme that occurs naturally in human

stomachs but sometimes becomes deficient. To remedy this imbalance and boost digestion and assimilation, readings for several hundred individuals suggest taking this enzyme (derived from animal stomachs) for short periods of time. Elixir or essence of lactated pepsin is a syrup form that is typically taken in water for its soothing effects:

> It will be found helpful to put small quantities of Essence of Lactated Pepsin in with the food or give it separate . . . This may be given at times when there apparently is more of the belching or tendency for the accumulations of same.   795-1

> The Pepsin is to act with the lacteals to produce more of the alkalin reaction . . .   1100-6

Keeping the diet MORE alkaline is clearly a key to staying on the sweet side of digestion, as the many commercials for relief of acidity attest. But when the stomach starts to rock and roll, we need relief in a hurry. Having some Cayce remedies on hand can shorten the wait and sweeten our dispositions at the same time.

Keeping the "Live" in Liver

The appropriately named liver joins with the kidneys and associated organs in a grand lifetime dance devoted to keeping the body as clean and detoxified as possible for as long as possible. The Cayce source regards the liver and kidneys as a kind of dynamic duo that may be balanced or ". . . unbalanced in the same manner, for . . . the liver is the opposite pole, as it were, from the kidneys . . . " (63-1)

Among the liver's hugely complex and varied functions are production of fluids used in digestion and creation of enzymes that neutralize toxins in the blood. It also makes hormones, breaks down fat, neutralizes bacteria and viruses, synthesizes proteins, and stores immune cells (macrophages), iron, and vitamins.

Dr. Richard Schulze refers to the liver as the ultimate energy and detoxification organ with good reason. One of its jobs is to convert carbohydrates into glucose and then store this in the body as a reserve energy supply. Another is to detoxify everything that passes through our mouths:

> Both the #1 and #2 causes of death are directly linked to the Liver. The #1 cause of death is Heart Attacks and Stroke caused by cholesterol blocking either coronary or cerebral arteries, killing the heart and the brain. IT'S THE LIVER'S JOB TO FILTER THIS CHOLESTEROL OUT OF YOUR BLOOD. The #2 cause of death is Cancer. Everyone now agrees that almost all cancers are caused by toxic carcinogenic chemicals in our food, water and air. These poisons get into our bloodstream, kill our cells, create tumors, cause cancer and kill us. IT'S THE LIVER'S JOB TO ELIMINATE THESE POISONS FROM OUR BLOOD.

Schulze goes on to say, "Most experts agree, from Constipation and Cataracts to even Cancer, many diseases start first with a sick, constipated Liver."[39]

In short, the liver is the body's first defensive barrier. However, it needs our support to do its job, especially with all the pollutants we ingest today. The good news, according to Cayce and others, is that with timely cleansing and nutrition, all but the sickest livers can be improved if not completely restored to health.

Cayce's literally thousands of references to the liver could easily fill a book, so only some highlights will be mentioned here. A factor common to all types of liver dysfunction is a surplus of toxins in the system. This is found to be the case in hepatitis, other infections, sluggish or torpid liver, cirrhosis, engorgement, and cases involving a lack of coordination between the liver and other organs. Toxicity is typically attributed to constipation and constipation to an overly acidic diet. The result is a backup in the liver and swelling of the organs around it, causing sluggishness, lack of coordination of all elimination functions, and a further backup of toxins.

---

[39]Richard Schulze, *Healing Liver and Gallbladder Disease Naturally* (California: Natural Healing Publications, 2003), 53–54.

When asked, in a case of hepatitis, what had caused the poisons in the system, Cayce responded:

> Inactivity of the liver and the eliminations through the regular channels, creating sedatives both in the kidney and in the activity of the gall ducts. 503-1

A person with torpid liver resulting from toxins coupled with "pressure" in the blood supply (probably hypertension) was warned that this needed to be quickly corrected. If not, some type of rheumatic, neuritic, or arthritic inflammation would arise, and " . . . it must also bring something of a hardening [cirrhosis] of the liver . . . " (331-1)

Clearly, a condition that is still at the "tendency" stage can be reversed:

> In the liver we find the greater seat of the troubles. This we find tends toward that of cirrhosis, though not at that stage as yet and may be brought to its proper functioning. 16-1

Cayce's therapies for the liver are always designed to reduce strain, gently detoxify the system, and provide whatever support is needed to regain proper functioning. Although treatments naturally vary with the scope and severity of the condition, several universally applicable ones stand out.

Many hundreds of readings advise the use of high enemas or colonic irrigations to relieve the pressure in the colon, reduce toxicity, and generally make it easier for the liver to function. Here are some typical instructions:

> . . . have a good hydrotherapist give a thorough but gentle colon cleansing—this possibly a week or two weeks apart. In the first waters, use salt and soda, in the proportions of a heaping teaspoonful of table salt and a level teaspoonful of baking soda dissolved thoroughly to each half gallon of water. In the last water use Glyco-Thymoline . . . to purify the system, in the proportions of a tablespoonful to the quart of water. 1745-4

Another outstanding recommendation is castor oil packs, which are more often placed over the liver area than any other location. These are low impact ways to stimulate the liver and step up its activity:

> We would increase the activity of the liver in its functioning, so as to bring about a better assimilation . . . through that of counterirritation externally, using those of the castor oil packs . . . and these should be kept up until there is a full activity from same . . . 18-2

Foremost among plants that have a stimulating and toning effect on the liver is ragweed, an herb regarded as especially beneficial to the liver and appendix. In Cayce's day this could be taken either as an ingredient in Simmons Liver Regulator, a product no longer on the market, or in a tea, tincture, or tonic for which specific directions were provided. One individual was advised to take " . . . either the ragweed {tea} or the Simmons' Liver Regulator, which is ragweed and licorice and a little senna." (304–18) To another, after providing tincture–making instructions, Cayce commented:

> And you have better than Simmons Liver Regulator for activity on the liver! This for anyone! This is the *best* of the vegetable compounds for activities of the liver.   369-12

Lastly is the matter of diet, which can be either a first cause or a remedy for liver distress. Cayce's advice, especially in acute conditions, is to stick to foods that are light but rich in nutrients, such as soup and vegetables. A person with torpid liver was told:

> Under the present condition, those of nourishing broths, salads or of such natures—that *rebuild* the system, as to satisfying of the appetite and of the stimulating of the system in a general manner. These should debar, then, anything that is for *heaviness only* in system.   325-28

Similarly, a reading for an individual with hepatitis advised:

> Do these, being mindful of the diet that there are not too much of starch or too great a quantity of meats taken; and we will bring this body to its normal reaction.   503-1

A frequent theme in advice for the liver is to keep the diet on the alkaline side and avoid highly acidic foods such as vinegar, meat, and carbohydrates:

> Keep in an alkalin reactory, but blood and nerve building. 209-1

> We would be mindful of the diet, that it is blood building and nerve building, but more tendency to those of alkaline than of acid.   63-1

As it does its dance in the body, the amazing liver is our lifetime partner in health. Whether we tango through life or have trouble getting off of the sofa is our choice.

No-Brainer Keys to Keeping Our Smarts

An especially common complaint, and perhaps even commoner joke, associated with aging is the incidence of "senior moments"—those quirky blips in the brain's normal retrieval process. It may be suddenly impossible to recall a name, a date, a phone number, an item on a shopping list, the location of the car keys, or the car. Whether, or how quickly, these symptoms of brain fog will worsen depends on many factors, but the specters of senile dementia and Alzheimer's disease are very real.

As with all looming fears, there are ways to keep these at bay or perhaps even exorcise them entirely. If Cayce's suggestions for doing so seem overly obvious, that's because they're so vital to our general health as well.

That the readings link a number of physical factors with both mental health and intelligence should come as no surprise. Like other cells in the body, brain cells require proper nourishment in order to function, or even survive:

. . . for the *life* of a brain *cell* is only according to the activity of a body physical and mental, and is *multiplied* according to the *activities* of same as related to the assimilation of resuscitating forces.   161-3

Both the nourishment of these vital tissues and the disposal of metabolic wastes (what Cayce called "used forces") are the tasks of the blood circulation. A sluggish flow can lead to physical discomfort, slowed mental processes, or both:

Q. What causes the pains in the head?
A. Lack of enough blood going there to supply the demand, using the force of the recuperative power to the brain in itself.   83-3

The lack of the blood force to supply needed tissue has an effect to the brain of making it tired when thinking . . .   3-1

Herbalist Dr. Schulze graphically fleshes out the picture of inadequate blood flow to the brain:

The brain, just like any organ, needs to assimilate nutrition and then eliminate waste. When the brain gets constipated, this blockage and subsequent back-up of waste, toxins, sludge, schmutz, goo, plaque, whatever you want to call it, causes your brain to get congested, which can then cause a thousand diseases from Alzheimer's, senility, eye and hearing disorders to paralysis.[40]

According to Cayce, a common factor in poor circulation is spinal misalignment, leading to "pressures" on certain nerves that originate along both sides of the vertebrae:

. . . in the brain forces, very good, yet the division in the blood

---

[40]Richard Schulze, *Dr. Schulze's 2011 Herbal Product Catalog* (Marina Del Rey, CA: American Botanical Pharmacy, 2011), 91.

supply and the subluxation in the first and third cervical . . . region
cause distress at times . . . to organs in the sensory system. 77-1

Such misalignments can result from injuries that may be quite long
standing or even from chronic emotional stress, as in a case attributed
to " . . . extreme nervous tension that overtaxed the system, as received
through the sensory forces, until the cells broke here at the 1st cervical."
(4097-1)

Cases of actual dementia in the readings are almost always linked to
nervous and circulatory system imbalances:

This condition is the form of hallucination dementia, and is produced, as we see, by a physical condition . . . that prevents the
normal flow of all blood to the brain in all its parts, for, as we see,
with a nerve structure debarred by pressure from normal action,
we have the same corresponding reaction in the brain proper.

173-1

Sure, dementia praecox is indicated, but it is from pressures—that
will respond. It will take time, but be patient, be persistent.

3441-1

A good preventive treatment, then, entails regular spinal adjustments,
the circulation boosters of one's choice, and, of course, a diet that will
keep the brain well nourished. An appointment with a skilled osteopath or chiropractor is an excellent place to start. Areas requiring special attention will probably include the extreme upper and lower spine.
Massage is especially important for those who are moving less often
and less vigorously, partly because it helps keep the blood flowing to
these vital areas:

The equalization of the circulation to minimize the strain on nerve
forces and brain (with the suggestions) should bring this body
back to normal.   151-1

For we can build with these, if there is the correct application of the Appliance and the massages, new brain and nerve tissue.

3496-1

A regular exercise program that includes walking (where possible) and stretching is the best way to stimulate the general circulation. Performing the head and neck exercise at least once a day will help keep the neck and shoulder muscles loose and the circulation to the brain flowing nicely. Brain cells, in particular, will benefit from a well-balanced diet that is high in vital nutrients:

> Do not overload the system with one element but balance the system better—more of that that is green and fresh and carrying more of the carbon in the system, not from meats but from vegetable matters, so that we will have the reaction to the body that will supply the energy of the system and give to the nerve forces, to the brain element, the elements necessary to replenish and not burn up energy in the system without replacing those conditions that will reproduce in the body, see?   257-1

Although it is not always possible to correct physical damage that has already taken place, the readings are generally optimistic, finding, even in some cases of actual dementia, that " . . . there might be added sufficient to the system in manners as to bring about nearer normal reactions for the body." (271-1)

Could "nearer normal" mean less senior moments? It's time to find out, even if it takes a lot of reminders.

A Farewell to Ulcers

Those prone to discomfort in the mid to upper abdominal region after meals or retiring may well be suffering from either ulcers or a pre-ulcerous condition. Hunger–like sensations such as gnawing, burning, and aching are signs of tissue erosion caused by our naturally acidic digestive juice. Erosion, lacerations or raw areas, and the discharge of pus can result, disturbing the lining of the stomach or duodenum—the uppermost part of the small intestine.

Why the body would begin to digest its own protective lining is a question with no pat answers. Both gastric and duodenal ulcers seem to stem from an imbalance between normal buffering mechanisms and acidic secretions, but the former variety develops later in life and is not linked to excess acid. Certain medications, such as aspirin, other NSAIDS, and possibly steroids, can be predisposing factors for some. Chronic nervous tension may or may not be involved. To compound the mystery, victims tend to experience periodic remission of symptoms or sometimes even spontaneous healing.

In all cases, the best way to temporarily relieve the symptoms of ulcers is by ingesting substances, such as milk, food, and antacids, which dilute and neutralize the acid. Medical management options depend on the severity of the condition.

The Edgar Cayce readings abound in helpful and hopeful suggestions for dealing with this perplexing and bothersome ailment. They contain detailed preventive and curative treatments given for over thirty-five individuals with ulcers and ulcerlike symptoms. Because the two types are treated similarly and are sometimes found in the same individual, they are considered here together.

Not surprisingly, an imbalance between the organs of assimilation and elimination is typically regarded as the primary cause. This, in turn, is attributed to or aggravated by factors such as dietary indiscretions, an overly taxed system, general weakness, congestion, flu, and constipation. A lack of proper secretions in the liver and other digestive organs is the end result, " . . . causing in the pyloric portion of the stomach a thickening or a caking in the wall of same . . . These cause a regurgitation, until there has been the back-flow of the hydrochloric into the pyloric portion of the stomach itself . . . And this, of course, in turn, by superacidity and the natural pressure, caused the great pains and the tendencies for the strains upon same." (1834-1)

Digestive imbalance sets the stage for ulcers in vulnerable individuals. An acute case of duodenal ulcers, or perhaps both types, is attributed simply to:

Overtaxation, and the general debilitation through the digestive system. Hence the flow of blood to the central portions of the body,

and taking away from head, see? With inflammation already in
head, the regurgitation or flowing back produces that of the congestion, see?   137-94

Another leading cause is chronic emotional stress in the form of nervous tension, negative attitudes, or anxiety. In these cases strain on the
nerves depletes the body to such an extent that the digestive process is
impaired. In one instance the resulting lack of muscle tone had actually
caused the stomach to tilt, setting the stage for irritation and the eventual development of ulcers.

An equally important factor is pressure on nerve ganglia governing
impulses to the elimination organs and digestive system. Spinal
misalignments are usually traced back to injuries, such as one that had
led to pressure just under the liver causing an adhesion. This, in turn,
was a major factor in the poor digestion, acid reflux, and lacerations
throughout the stomach area.

Although conditions such as the above had not yet evolved into
ulcers, others were about as acute as possible:

Yes—the body is *almost* as near in an explosive condition as the
materials they are handling here.   1970-1

Initial treatments in all cases focus primarily on alleviating symptoms so the rebuilding process can begin. The first step is always to coat
and soothe the intestinal lining so that raw or infected areas are able to
heal. A preferred way to accomplish this is to drink saffron tea, elm
water, or both throughout the day. These demulcent beverages are intended to " . . . act with the gastric juices as to relieve those burning
sensations as continue to act with the system." *(5641-1)* In speaking of
elm water, which is made by stirring a pinch of the powdered bark into
a glass of water, one reading wryly noted: " . . . It will be as slime, of
course, but this is what's needed in the alimentary canal." (5216-1)

Another way to soothe the intestinal tract is by ingesting small doses
of olive oil " . . . so that the activity to the gastric flow of the stomach is
as a food value to the whole of the intestinal system." (732-1) At the
same time, it is important to reduce acidity through the use of gentle

alkalizing agents and digestive aids such as limewater, cinnamon water, Glyco-Thymoline, lactated pepsin, Al-Caroid, and bismuth preparations. Priority is also given in many cases to relieving pressure on the colon through colonic irrigations, enemas, and gentle laxatives such as Milk of Magnesia, Castoria, and Eno Salts. Specific treatment sequences ensure that the body is not overly stressed at any given time.

Cayce's dietary advice, which not surprisingly appears in virtually every case, varies with the severity of symptoms. In acute situations, the diet given is extremely limited and often semi-liquid at first to avoid further strain on the system. The menu in the explosive situation mentioned above consisted of Concord grapes, junket (a digestive enzyme source), and crackers. After a week to ten days other digestible items could be added, such as milk, cheese, beef juice, cooked vegetables, liver, and liver extract. Other foods often recommended for easy assimilation include yogurt, buttermilk, malted milk, eggnog, cooked cereals, whole grain breads, arrowroot, chicken broth, citrus juices, raw vegetables, and vegetable juices. Foods and beverages specifically banned include fried foods, white bread, white potatoes, spaghetti, cheese, sodas, and beer.

Spinal adjustments are advised in many of these cases to remove the effects of injuries and speed healing by relaxing and balancing the nerves. Other treatments sometimes mentioned include castor oil packs, massage, grape poultices, hydrotherapy, electrotherapy, rest, spending time outdoors, and positive attitudes. A few readings strongly advised against having surgery, at least at that time.

Reports indicating whether these treatments were followed are few although the wife of case 5618, a medical doctor, testified: " . . . Mr. Cayce also diagnosed the case of my husband . . . for what seemed like an incurable stomach trouble of long standing with most satisfactory results; which condition had refused to yield to his own treatment or that of other physicians . . . "

The readings themselves are highly optimistic that following their advice consistently over time can lead to a complete cure—perhaps even a digestive system that Superman would admire: " . . . But with the use of these properties as indicated—Well, in six months he can eat nails if he likes!" (732-1)

Who could wish for a stronger stomach than that?

Kidney TLC

As with other major organs, our kidneys can be damaged to the point of temporary malfunctions or worse. Moreover, much as we'd like to avoid taking responsibility, most kidney glitches are not caused by accidents or bad genes but are the cumulative results of our own lifestyle choices. The body's blood filtration system is actually rather delicate and can respond quite dramatically to neglect. Those who have ever had a kidney stone learned this lesson the hard way. Life is much more pleasant when we treat our hard-working kidneys with the care they deserve.

These two bean-shaped organs, each about the size of one's palm, are located on either side of the spine. It's a good thing there are two of them because filtering out water (95%) and other dissolved substances (5%) and monitoring the blood's acid/alkaline balance are full-time jobs. If one kidney poops out, the other valiantly carries on, but it's lonelier and riskier that way. That 5% of metabolic waste products excreted by the kidneys to pass through the ureters and then the bladder is really pretty varied, consisting as it does of minerals, urea, uric acid, sugars, creatine, creatinine, ammonia, and sometimes more hazardous wastes depending on one's state of health.

In fact, our kidneys, along with what comes out of them, can mirror our health, or lack of it, quite accurately. No training in urinalysis is needed to note when the urine seems extra concentrated and to deduce that this indicates dehydration. A burning sensation while urinating often means infection. Aches and pains in kidney locations can mean infection or stones. Chronic kidney disease is often associated with on-going conditions like diabetes or hypertension.

How do kidney problems start? To begin with, they simply become slightly overtaxed by working under unusually stressful conditions. There may be a bout with illness, poor dietary choices, dehydration, sluggish eliminations, circulatory imbalances, an overly toxic system, or all of the above.

When such imbalances are corrected, the kidneys bounce back usually as good as new, but if any become chronic, that's another story. The mineral sedimentation that leads to kidney stones, according to Cayce and other sources, can result from an overly acidic diet. The readings target red meat, refined carbohydrates, vinegar, and possibly carbonated drinks as dietary culprits. High blood pressure can eventually clog and scar the filtering system's tiny parts, leading to irreparable damage. Here, again, diet can be part of the problem. Herbalist Dr. Richard Schulze puts it this way:

> Your kidneys and bladder may be congested, overloaded and plugged because your food program is too high in Animal Foods. This causes hyper-cholesterolemia (high cholesterol levels) which in turn causes hypertension (high blood pressure). High blood pressure causes almost half of all kidney disease.
>
> Your kidneys have a much harder time filtering out thick fatty blood than filtering out thinner blood. This is just basic physics. Try pouring water through a coffee filter. Now try pouring ice cream or cheese through the same coffee filter. Not very easy, is it?[41]

When our filtration system breaks down, so does the entire body—so we don't want to go there. Instead, we'll focus on helpful tips for kidney care and maintenance taken from the hundreds of readings on the subject. Cayce's tone is generally extremely optimistic about the effectiveness of noninvasive treatments, systematic cleanses, and improvement of general health. Dr. Schulze agrees with this course of action:

> The only reason your kidneys are failing is because the blood they are trying to filter is more like a toxic sludge. If you clean up your lifestyle, your food program, flush out your elimination organs (especially your Bowel, your Liver and Gallbladder and of course your

---

[41]Richard Schulze, *25 Ways to Have the Cleanest Kidneys* (California: Natural Healing Publications, 2004), 21.

Kidneys) your kidneys and your body will heal itself.[42]

Cayce's tactics for reducing kidney stress are gentle and effective. All can help support optimal function whether one is under a doctor's care or not. Some are clearly preventive, as well.

A light, easily digested diet that prevents further strain on the entire excretory system is a must. (In cases of kidney stones, make that diet liquid or semiliquid.) The readings especially favor fruits and vegetables at such times. These are best accompanied by blood and body–building choices such as whole grain cereals, beef juice, eggnog, red wine with dark bread, and plenty of water between meals. At least one person was told categorically to avoid carbonated beverages. Another was advised:

> Let the diet be not meats of the heavy or greasy nature. Much of the lentils, beans and food values of that nature. Much fruit, and little of vinegar or of those elements carrying acetic acid producing juices. That is, little tomatoes, no pickles unless it's sweet.
>
> 427-2

Since pressure on certain vertebrae, caused by accident or other stress, can slow circulation to the kidneys, having a spinal adjustment every so often is a good idea. The part(s) of the spine where corrections are needed will vary with the individual:

> A balance in digestion and elimination, as would be created by correction . . . in dorsal and cervical region, and with the acidity relieved in system, the strain on kidneys will be removed. 340-5

Various types of hot packs and poultices are helpful in easing discomfort, drawing out toxins, and increasing circulation in affected areas. These are usually to be placed over the lower back, abdomen, or both areas. Hot salt packs receive most frequent mention, sometimes in combination with Glyco–Thymoline stupes, mullein stupes, or a combi-

---

[42]Ibid., 33.

nation of mutton tallow, turpentine spirits, and camphor spirits. This latter formula can easily be worked into congested areas as part of a massage and then kept warm to induce relaxation:

> These will relieve the pressure and strain.   632-5

> . . . making for something of a counterirritant, externally, to those tendencies of the kidneys for their inflammatory conditions that arise at times; thus producing—through the activity of the bladder and the regular system as it attempts to eliminate—a preventative from these conditions becoming centralized or localized . . .   632-6

The use of light diuretics will step up the flow of urine and speed the removal of any accumulated toxins. This is an especially good idea if infection is suspected or known to be present. One of Cayce's favorites for this purpose is watermelon seed tea:

> This will clarify those conditions that cause reactions in the kidneys and bladder, for, the lack of eliminations and the slowing up of the circulation causes a greater quantity of drosses to be held in the system, and these need to be eliminated from the body.
>   More will be eliminated through using this stimuli for the kidney activity than in most any way.   1695-2

Even Coca–Cola, though without the fizz, is found to be a helpful diuretic for some:

> Do take coca cola occasionally as a drink for the activity of the kidneys, but do not take it with carbonated water. Buy or have the syrup prepared and add plain water to this. Take about ½ oz. or 1 oz. of the syrup and add plain water. This to be taken about every other day with or without ice. This will aid in purifying the kidney activity and bladder and will be better for the body.   5097-1

Finally, and first among beverages, is water itself. Although the body's daily liquid requirement can be taken in a number of forms (teas, juices, soups, etc.), it is important that much of that liquid be, simply, water. Although health authorities disagree on how much, the readings favor six to eight glasses daily and often comment:

> Well to drink *always plenty* of water, before meals and after meals . . .   311-4

The water thing is a stumbling block for many before something like a kidney stone sounds the alarm, that is. Pain is such a powerful motivator. It's much more fun to become a water worshiper and feel those kidneys jumping for joy. Why not give yours a little TLC today?

Keeping the Beat: Help for Skipping Hearts

Arrhythmia, or irregular heartbeat, can have a number of causes, varies in severity, and may or may not require carefully monitored treatment. This is a huge oversimplification of an extremely complex topic that occupies physicians in a very big way. The bottom line is that heart disease is serious business, and symptoms are expected to worsen.

Since only thirteen readings, many only in passing, concern themselves with this disorder, Cayce's contribution is small. However, his comments shed a great deal of light on possible origins and on early, or even preventive, treatment.

To begin with, most of the recipients of these readings were given the encouraging news that their irregular beats did not indicate an actual heart condition—as yet. Rather, they were signs of systemic imbalances that needed to be corrected before they worsened and did, indeed, do permanent damage. The disturbing symptoms typically were indicative of the body's attempt to equalize the circulation between the heart, lungs, liver, and kidneys. Specific stress-inducing factors, such as poor elimination, indigestion, toxicity, and spinal misalignments, were often involved:

> This is rather of the liver, *not* of the heart, though the congestion in the liver makes the quick pulsation and the irregularity there.
>   1521-4

. . . no organic disturbance, but an erratic—or quite a variation in the—heartbeat itself at times.   2797-1

. . . rather a sympathetic condition to those disturbances through eliminating channels.   462-17

The system's attempting to adjust itself to the *proper* coordination of extremities of the body.   264-11

It's a reflex condition in the nervous system . . . as well as a general nervous condition.   2946-5

The blood supply shows a slowing of circulation, while the pulsation at times quickens—or becomes irregular.   2951-1

What stands out in these cause–and–effect descriptions is the repeated message that this imbalance may often be at least largely correctible. Cayce basically told these people that their hearts would stop skipping beats when the internal stresses affecting their circulatory flow were relieved. However, prompt action was needed before the condition worsened, especially in the two or three more serious cases.

Although arrhythmia was not the primary concern that prompted these readings, treatments are surprisingly consistent. A series of osteopathic adjustments and/or massages is recommended in eleven cases to release nerve impingements and relax the muscles around them. These corrections are regarded as central to healing in cases where a lack of coordination between the cerebrospinal and autonomic nervous systems is impairing what Cayce called the "deeper circulation" between the heart and other vital organs.

Aids to digestion and elimination are found in ten cases—a figure that goes even higher when diet is included. The main internal substances, with none mentioned more than twice, are Acigest, Calcios, Castoria, and mullein tea. External cleansing measures include colonics, enemas, castor oil packs, and hydrotherapy measures such as fume baths.

Dietary instructions, given in nine cases, are unanimous in preferring foods that are alkaline forming, laxative, and highly nourishing at the same time. This requires a strong emphasis on vegetables, such as watercress, beet tops, and anything else one would put in a salad, as well as all types of raw juices. Fish, fowl, lamb, and meat juices are the preferred proteins. Whole grain cereals, gelatin, egg yolks, nuts, fruit juices, and light wines are all sometimes recommended. Prohibited items include all fried foods, red meat, carbonated drinks, white potatoes, and in one case, chocolate.

Electrotherapy treatments, mentioned in five cases, vary too much to suggest a definite pattern though both the Wet Cell and Radio-Active Appliance are each recommended twice. Several of these individuals were advised to take it easy physically until conditions improved. According to some of their reports, finding time to really rest was, indeed, a major hurdle.

Reports received in several cases were sketchy but generally positive in proportion to how quickly and consistently the treatments were followed. In at least one instance, arrhythmia ceased to be a problem.

Bringing Up Beautiful Babies

There is no denying that a healthy baby is a beautiful baby, regardless of how the family genes are dealt out. We also know that good health maximizes anyone's chance of success in life, so the quality of nurturing during infancy and early childhood is vitally important. Since how this translates into daily choices seems so complex these days, it is helpful to focus on creating a wholesome, and perhaps simpler, climate for raising young children where the gentle, commonsense attention to detail that keeps babies thriving really doesn't change very much. That's the wisdom on this topic that plays out in the course of several hundred Cayce files.

Assembling the building blocks for a vibrantly healthy child actually begins well before conception, so we'll start there. It is well known that difficulty conceiving can indicate physical issues and that the healthier one is at the time of conception, the better for mother and child. Women who asked about how to prepare were typically told to focus first on their health through a high quality diet, appropriate exercise, and so forth. A woman of twenty-five was counseled to balance her activity and rest, receive a series of colonics and osteopathic treatments, and improve her diet:

> Beware of sugars, but let those sugars as are taken be most of fruit and of nuts, and the rest in . . . those as bring forth the vibrations of the vegetable kingdom. 136-83

The importance of aligning the spine is echoed in a reading for a thirty-two-year-old woman who asked whether weight or flexibility was a more important issue during childbirth:

> Pliability of the body. Thus the greater preparation *this* body may make, or *most* bodies for that matter, is to be under the care of a competent osteopath through the period of gestation; not a chiropractor but an osteopath! 457-8

Those who were already pregnant were given similar, though usually more extensive, advice. When the above woman, who received readings during her pregnancies two and four years later, wanted to know whether adjustments were still appropriate, the categorical response was:

> Practically always advisable during pregnancy. 457-9

> If mothers would only know that a good gynecologist of the osteopathic school would save more mothers from hard labor! 457-14

Similar advice was offered in a reading for a twenty-eight-year-old woman that advised plenty of moderate exercise in the open while warning against strenuous exertion:

> We would occasionally—once in two weeks—have a thorough relaxing of the system osteopathically, for the *bodily* forces to *adjust* themselves to the *development* of those conditions with the body.

As should be understood, of course, these should not be for corrections, other than *assisting* the body in correcting its new positions—especially through those areas from the first of the dorsals to the pelvic portions, of course, and the coccyx area. 23-14

Two superior forms of pain relief, during pregnancy and beyond, are osteopathy and massage, especially when the effect of medication on the fetus is considered. One reading recommended spinal rubs with olive oil and myrrh to relieve headaches and provide other benefits for a twenty-two-year-old new mother:

This will be found strengthening and beneficial toward the entity gaining its physical strength, and in the correction of those conditions necessary to bring about the healing properties in these portions of body by that increased circulation to these parts. 136-60

Throughout the course of pregnancy, nutrition remains of vital importance for the developing needs of mother and child. Typical instructions focus on foods high in both nutrients and fiber, such as fruits, vegetables, whole grains, and the lighter proteins:

That which carries sufficient, as indicated . . . , of the general nourishment for the blood and nerve building forces of the body. Not meats, but sufficient proteins—of course—to keep the strength and vitality of the whole general system.   301-8

A reading for a thirty-six-year-old woman gave similar guidelines while warning against more than small amounts of coffee, tea, and alcohol:

No fermentations are good for system under condition, save as necessary for digestion and blood building for both.   780-5

Taking supplemental sources of vitamins A, D, and iron (in Cayce's day often through a product known as Codiron) is considered important in some readings. Many also indicate a need for extra calcium from limes, dairy products, and a super digestible source known as Calcios:

> Rather than the calcium tablets, use *Calcios*. This is better assimi-
> lated, and does not leave as much dregs to become a hardship to
> the liver *and* the kidneys, and works better with the activities of
> the system as related to the cod liver oil for better development.
>   23-14

Cayce's dietary advice for just after birth continues to focus on the
mother because of the importance of high quality breast milk. A twenty-
five-year-old woman anticipating delivery in two weeks was told:

> If the body is to care for the baby itself, as it *should*—all normal
> ones should—these should consist of those that will make for . . .
> the *development* of those foods for the child—see? These would
> consist more of those of vegetables that carry the proteins, the
> irons, and those of such nature, with plenty of milk and plenty of
> cheese and of such natures that supply the bone and blood build-
> ing forces as may be supplied through the nourishment as for self
> and as for the offspring.   301-6

In a similar vein, the mother of a three-month-old was advised to:

> Drink plenty of milk as long as the body nurses the baby, see?
> This supplies not only calcium for self, but will also supply a much
> better and much more even diet to be *with* the supplying for the
> body of the baby.   301-7

In cases where the flow or quality of breast milk seems inadequate,
an upgrading of the mother's diet is in order. One new mother in this
situation was given a list of foods to emphasize that included dry milk,
Ovaltine, oatmeal, and other vitamin-rich cereals. The mother of a
seven-week-old was advised to balance sources of protein and vitamin
D with plenty of alkaline-forming foods and to go easy on fats and
sugar. Precautions regarding sweets, vinegar, and other acidic foods are
found in other readings as well. Warnings regarding fat were repeated

in a reading for a two-day-old infant:

> As has been indicated, *fats* are the most detrimental to all infants
> in this developing stage.   1208-2

The question of how long to nurse is, of course, treated individually. The mother of a three-month-old was advised to do so as long as the process continued to be beneficial and free of strain for her and her child. In the case of a one-year-old who was obviously eating plenty of solid food, the nursing was still considered beneficial until the teeth were better developed.

At times when the breast milk did not meet the baby's needs, Cayce did not hesitate to recommend supplementing or even replacing it temporarily while the mother's health improved. Signs of poor quality milk in these cases included indigestion, colic, failure to thrive, and congestion. For infants of two months or less, the usual choice was a prepared formula such as one made by Carnation or a product called Mellin's Food. The diets of babies from three months or so could be boosted with small amounts of regular foods, such as strained oatmeal, Gerber's vegetable juices, and fresh orange juice.

Dietary guidelines for older babies, whether still nursing or not, branch out considerably, though they continue to focus on high quality nutrition in a simple, easily digested form. Foods recommended for a six-month-old include milk and overcooked oatmeal. Readings for two one-year-olds mention Mellin's Food, milk, Gerber vegetables, tomato juice, bacon, egg yolk, and vegetable soups. Blood building diets given for two one-and-a-half-year-olds include citrus and pineapple juices, coddled egg yolks, Gerber vegetable juices, rice, milk, vegetables, liver, and Zwieback. Foods advised for two twenty-month-olds include dry and cooked cereal with cream, meat juices, broths, vegetables, vegetable juices, cooked apples, and yogurt. Diets in cases where congestion is present center on alkaline foods with high liquid content. Overfeeding and sugar are not approved:

> Do not give too much sugars! *These* are what have upset the whole
> of the digestive system!   1208-12

> *Do not* give sugar in *any* form other than from fruit or vegetables,
> until after he is at least eighteen months old! . . . Sugars will make
> for the easy assimilation or activity of cold, for it produces acid—
> which makes the body susceptible to changes.   1208-6

Another facet of healthy development for babies (as well as people in
general) is plenty of time in the open, so long as cold, dampness, and
drafts don't worsen any congestion. For infants, fresh air and indirect
sunlight are sufficient, while for more developed babies, some direct
light is beneficial for growth. In the case of a five–month–old, morning
or afternoon time spent in dry sand was found to be beneficial. Sunlight was highly recommended for a nine–month–old:

> . . . For, the ultra-violet forces from the sun's rays will not only
> strengthen the superficial circulation but will strike deeper into the
> body . . .
>   Hence, to give the body sun baths at specific periods through
> the day would be well at all times through this particular period of
> development.   305-1

Massage is another way to enliven the circulation, strengthen the
body, keep the skin hydrated, and perhaps even act as a form of preventive medicine. Under normal circumstances, as in the case of a three-
month–old, cocoa butter and olive oil were typically endorsed:

> After the bath of morning, it would be well occasionally to gently
> massage the whole of the cerebrospinal system—one time with
> Olive Oil, the next time with Cocoa Butter.
>   These, as we find, are the better for the developments through
> those periods of the body's activity for the next six to eight months.
>   2015-4

Spinal massage with olive oil was a treatment of choice for a twenty-
two–month–old whose poor diet had led to anemia, low weight, acidity,
and infection. A reading for an eighteen–month–old found that cocoa
butter massage would actually help to ward off congestion:

For the better development of the circulation through the head
and through the upper portion of the body, each evening when
ready for retirement—for at least a period of ten days to two
weeks—we would massage with cocoa-butter along the upper
dorsal and cervical area. The vibrations of this with the muscular
system and with the blood supply will prevent the congestions in
the area, that would make for disturbances.   773-2

In situations where congestion had already taken hold, camphor liniments were usually preferred. For a thirteen–month–old with congestion and fever, Cayce recommended rubbing camphorated olive oil into
her spine, chest, throat, and feet. Readings for a fifteen–month–old advised a solution of camphor spirits, turpentine spirits, and mutton tallow for this purpose.

The subject of congestion is huge, with poor diet and resulting indigestion and acidity cited as primary causes. A common recommendation for digestive troubles is limewater, an alkaline mineral solution
sometimes accompanied by cinnamon water. Small amounts of limewater given just after nursing or added to formula, milk, or juice are
often considered the remedy of choice even in cases of infant colic. The
mother of a three-week-old with this problem was advised:

But, as we find, it would be more helpful to add a teaspoonful of
limewater to each quantity of milk as nursed, see? Necessarily
this would be diluted; not put in the milk but diluted and given
afterwards . . . This {hiccoughing} is natural, and—with the limewater—will be eliminated.   928-1

A specific for congestion and related difficulties is a senna–based
stomach sweetener and gentle elimination aid known as Castoria. This
syrupy liquid is best given in tiny doses of a drop or two at a time over
the course of a day:

Colds should be worked off with Castoria, which sweetens the
stomach and makes for the better digestion.   1208-6

Aid the eliminations; for there is an upsetting of the gastric forces in the stomach from which this cough emanates—see? Hence the sweetening of the gastric forces with properties combined with senna, in small quantities, would be helpful—as in Castoria—for keeping an even balance. Small quantities given often are much more effective than larger quantities given to simply produce eliminations. See?   314-2

Milk of Magnesia, another gentle elimination aid, is sometimes advised as well. Miniscule amounts of Glyco-Thymoline are also widely recommended for congested babies. For respiratory relief, a prescription item made from an onion-like bulb known as Syrup of Squill is often employed.

Incidentally, teething woes are usually to be addressed by rubbing diluted Ipsab solutions into the gums:

We would find that a weakened solution of Ipsab for the gums would tend to reduce the pressure and make for normalcy in the salivary glands, as well as strengthening the tissue in mouth. This should be reduced at least half, and the gums massaged with a tuft of cotton with same. This also adds to the amount of saline, calcium and iodine, for the activity of the glands in mouth and throat.   299-2

Last, but most vital to any budding beauty, is the nurturing effect of constructive attitudes. Negative emotions such as resentment are especially detrimental, or as one reading for a very new mother warned: " . . . And *anger!* Keep from *anger!"* (1208-2) The best advice for any parent is always to:

Keep the body as near physically fit as possible. Keep happy. Keep glad. This makes for better conditions for self and for body dependent on self.   301-8

Putting a Stop to Stuttering

Most people stumble while speaking from time to time. Like tripping on the sidewalk, stuttering and its milder variant stammering only become problems when they happen persistently. We're even supposed to laugh when cartoon characters like Porky Pig try to talk, suggesting that a certain amount of stuttering in children is considered cute and endearing.

However, the charm quickly fades when the hesitations and spasmodic repetitions persist in children or develop later in life. Twelve individuals were sufficiently concerned about these symptoms to request readings for themselves or their children. Although the severity of symptoms is unknown, these readings are remarkably consistent in their diagnoses and treatments. Cayce's persistent optimism about the effectiveness of these simple measures is just as impressive.

The subjects of these readings ranged in age, so far as this was given, from three to forty-three, including one teenager and five children age nine and younger. The central problem found by Cayce in most, if not all, of these cases was a nervous imbalance, described as a lack of coordination between the cerebrospinal and sympathetic nervous systems. The original cause of this imbalance, when given, was most typically an injury of external origin. A twenty-nine-year-old man who had suffered a concussion in an automobile accident two months earlier was told:

> Rather has there been an upsetting of the system from violent influences from without, so that in many portions of the system there is the necessity for a coordinating throughout the cerebrospinal system . . .   416-5

Similarly, a reading for a thirty-seven-year-old man explained that the effects of an accident combined with congestion had caused distress in the sympathetic system and led to a number of symptoms:

> These produce this humming in the ears, the tendency for the body to stutter, or to have to think before words are spoken, and the reflexes in the eye.   99-1

Accidents were also cited in readings for children who had trouble mastering speech. The first cause in one case was described as a slight wrenching of the spine, apparently due to a fall, that had led to nerve impingements that were affecting the voice. The stammering of a five-year-old girl was attributed to long-standing spinal pressures and nerve system imbalance resulting from a fall at the age of eighteen months.

In several older individuals, the nerves were affected, at least in part, by shock, nervous tension, or taxation. A forty-three-year-old war veteran was told:

> As we find, then, these conditions were produced *from* nervous shock, and the reaction caused the ganglia to become dissipated . . . when there is the attempt to coordinate the nerves between the central nervous system and the sensory.   2705-1

The causes were different but the effects apparently quite similar in the case of a nervous and frustrated thirteen-year-old girl:

> Then, the condition is an abnormalcy in the imaginative or psychic force of the body, as related to the coordinating of the active forces between the sympathetic and cerebrospinal impulses that go to make up those forces in responding to that in the speech.
>   605-1

And a thirty-nine-year-old woman suffering from nervous taxation affecting her entire body was told:

> Functioning of the organs of the sensory system, these show retraction at times; strain as is caused to the eye from nerve, to the ear from nerve, to the speech, and the stuttering or the choking, and inability to speak the things that are thought in the body at times. Lack of perfect coordination throughout, from nerve retractions and nerve debilitation in the system.   4409-1

In most of these cases the readings are extremely clear and consistent about the areas of the spine affecting the speech. The mid to upper cervical or neck vertebrae and the upper dorsal (thoracic today) are the usual areas of focus. The parents of a four-year-old boy who asked about the causes of stuttering were given the following explanation:

In the body-forces, as we have oft indicated through this channel, each portion of the organism of the body is controlled by coordination of the sympathetic and cerebrospinal nervous system. The connections for the auditory as well as the vocal forces of the body derive their impulse from the 3rd cervical, as well as the 3rd, 4th and 5th dorsal.   1788-13

A reading for one of the accident victims gives further details about the effects of an upper cervical injury:

From the upper cervical area there is produced the tendency for dizziness, forgetfulness, irritations that cause singing and drumming in the ear, affectations to the speech [stuttering], and even to the vision at times. All of these effects are disturbing factors, not by impingements but rather engorgements in the 3rd, 5th and 2nd cervicals; especially where these make for their associations with the divisions to the vagus nerves.   416-5

The occasional references to the vagus nerves in this group of readings should be of special interest to those who practice spinal manipulation. This is the name for the tenth pair of cranial nerves arising from the medulla or brain stem. These branch out to various organs and apparently to the speech apparatus as well.

Naturally there are other contributing factors to be addressed in these cases, including mental attitudes, congestion, and karmic situations. However, these are all over the map, as might be expected.

Cayce's treatment strategies also vary, although spinal manipulation is consistently advised in almost every case. Here is a typical protocol, provided for the four-year-old mentioned above:

Hence it is necessary, very patiently but very systematically, to reduce—osteopathically—those tendencies of the body to over-supply energies to the vocal cords . . .

And these as we find, while requiring some time and some patience, will relieve stuttering; that is, the osteopathic corrections, with special reference to the connecting centers in the lymph patches, the emunctory activity and circulation, from those areas indicated in the spine *[cervical and thoracic]*, should assist the body in correcting those tendencies existent.   1788-13

Gentler substitutes for actual manipulation of vertebrae were indicated where needed. For the woman with nervous taxation, electric vibrator massage was the preferred method. Massage with oil, in one case along with spinal adjustments, was the treatment advised for two of the younger children.

As a broad category of treatment, electrotherapy is important enough to receive mention in many of these cases. Although the method used varies from one case to the next, all share the central goal of revitalizing the circulation.

Some degree of mental effort, through determination, prayer, Bible reading, forgiveness, or a willingness to accept hands-on healing, is a treatment element in a number of cases. The girl in her teens was encouraged to work consciously with her attitudes:

And be mindful that the body overcomes this tendency of becoming frustrated; and this lisping and stammering will disappear.
605-3

A very interesting exchange took place between Cayce and the one person who received no physical treatment advice:

Q. Is it possible through this approach to tell me how I may overcome the stammering, or is it purely physical?
A. The body can deal with any situation effectively if it trusts in the ideal manner. Not in self, no—never, but in Him, who is the way and the truth and the light.   3245-1

A calm assurance that a consistent course of treatment will get results comes through these readings loud and clear:

And the body should be near normal.   416-5

. . . these conditions may be eliminated entirely from the system.
                                                                    1788-13

Several glowing reports show the accuracy of Cayce's predictions.
The auto accident victim's stuttering cleared up after the first few osteopathic treatments. The parents of one injured child later shared that:
" . . . Her stuttering is very much improved . . . " (2015-8) and still later
that it had stopped entirely. In another report, a delighted parent commented:

> She seems to be less nervous, and her stammering has almost
> completely disappeared. I feel she has made great progress. We
> have been very consistent in her treatments.   1490-3

The bottom line is that stuttering and stammering can be stopped.
The only place they should be allowed to continue is, perhaps, in gentle
humor.

Taking the Punch out of Rheumatism and Neuritis

Creaky, inflamed joints take the joy out of living for untold numbers
of people, making them feel old before their time. Although often regarded as one of those inevitable tolls taken by aging, rheumatic disease can also afflict the middle-aged and even the young with equally
crippling effects.

Rheumatism is actually a blanket term for a group of painful joint
and muscle conditions that includes rheumatoid arthritis, bursitis, and
neuritis. In RA, chronic swelling and joint inflammation are accompanied by muscle spasms and often result in joint deformities. Bursitis is
an inflammation of a fluid-filled sac protecting a shoulder or hip joint
while neuritis is a nerve inflammation that can lead to degenerative
changes.

Many symptoms of osteoarthritis are attributed, at least in part, to
the aftereffects of injury or even to occupational stress. However, the
root causes of the rheumatoid variety are considered medically unknown. Neither is a puzzle for the Edgar Cayce readings, which offer a

clearer understanding of both causes and treatment of rheumatic disease.

This study of about one quarter of the over four hundred available documents boils down to fifty–eight pertinent readings given for thirty-six individuals who ranged in age from thirteen to seventy-two. The rheumatic and sometimes also neuritic symptoms in these cases affected many different areas of the body, including knees, wrists, feet, hips, fingers, arms, back, shoulder joints, elbows, and neck.

Cayce's descriptions of how rheumatic conditions originate paint a scenario of inadequately eliminated waste products trapped in the bloodstream until they lodge in vulnerable areas of the body. Typically, this process begins with infection, sluggish elimination, or both. In cases of infection, congestion and inflammation overload the body's systems and organs of elimination with toxins. This hinders the circulation of blood and lymphatic fluid throughout the body and to the extremities, in particular. In cases of poor elimination, an overly acidic diet and poor hydration progress gradually toward chronic constipation and indigestion. Again, the result is toxins in the circulation and an increased susceptibility to congestion and infection.

Impaired circulation slows both nutrient supply and removal of crystallized minerals and uric acid. If such an imbalance is not corrected, muscles and joints in the affected areas begin to stiffen, leading to pain and inflammation of tissues and associated nerve endings. This can easily become chronic, requiring much greater effort to reverse the process later.

Toxicity obviously plays a central role in rheumatic disorders. This can lead to a dangerous system–wide infection known as toxemia, as seen in almost half of these cases:

> . . . the drosses from non-eliminated used forces are the greater disturbing elements in the body, and the nerve strain under which the body exerts same . . .   121-1

> . . . the toxins being carried in the blood supply . . . are left in the tissue and sinew in portions of the body, and cause pain to the body at times, in the form of contraction of the muscular forces over certain portions of the system . . .   159-1

Q. What causes the trouble in the knee?
A. That of absorption of poisons in the system, irritation by injuries as have been received from time to time, and of centralization of poisons as are left in system carried by circulation, and the anterior or capillary circulation becoming slow . . .   265-5

References to poor elimination, both in general and in greater detail, are found in a similar number of cases:

Poor eliminations through the system, and the change, as it were—retractions throughout the body.   25-5

. . . lack of proper eliminations of the poisons of the system, as well as that of drosses being carried.   119-1

Q. Why does pain continue in my left foot?
A. The effect of poisons in the system that have not been entirely eliminated.   257-133

Q. Do I have Arthritis?
A. No. These effects are from the poor eliminations, and there is not an indication in the blood stream nor in the acidity of the system of these being arthritis. It is more of the rheumatic effect from the strain upon the kidneys owing to the activities, and thus producing uric acid in the system.   313-10

Q. What are the causes of the joints being so sore, and what will relieve them?
A. Increase the eliminations. These are the effects of pressure, by poisons in system not eliminated, and radiate from those centers and plexuses as are governed by the mesenteric system. 325-17

Q. What is the cause of the rheumatism?
A. The effect of these conditions as are given, coming from the kidneys in their activity.   462-2

Spinal lesions and misalignments appear as causative factors in about one fourth of these cases. The readings attribute these to either external factors such as falls and injuries or to internal pressures caused by elimination or digestive issues:

Q. What is the cause of the queer snapping in the joints when the body moves at times, and what may be done to correct this?
A. Those strains that are on the nerve system, where the blood supply—in its assimilation, as comes from joints themselves—would create the condition as body is being warned of. Rheumatic, arthritic, and such conditions, would be a result . . .   295-2

Widespread congestion and infection are found with similar frequency. Either can move beyond the respiratory system into other sensitive areas of the body:

Hence we may have catarrh of the head, of the throat, of the stomach, of the intestines, or it may become so distributed as to become known as other names in the effect produced upon the joint, or the sinew, or the muscle, or of tissue in various portions of the system . . . here we find it more active in the action of the lymph with the lymphatic circulation being depressed by same . . . in affecting most the sinew or the muscular retraction in body. 92-1

Similarly, a reading for a sixteen-year-old boy attributes difficulties with walking to the aftereffects of rheumatic fever:

. . . hence the inability of the lymphatic centers in extremities to coordinate with the nerve and tissue of the body in those portions of the system. Hence under knees, in arms, in feet, in the locomotaries we find those have become taut, and the centers do not function in their normal way and manner.   25-1

Impaired circulation, digestive system imbalances, and spinal pressures are often related factors, as in the case of a thirty-nine-year-old man with toxemia and rheumatism tendencies:

Q. What causes pain in under side of left arm, wrist, and ankle
joints?
A. Poor circulation to the extremities of the body, through pressures in the area adjoining the brachial plexus, and reflex to the
lumbar plexus: and becomes accentuated by the pressure produced in colon area, that makes reflex actions to all of these tendencies. Hence *reducing* the pressure!   306-3

Mineral imbalance can be another contributing factor, as in the case
of a fifty–one–year–old woman with both rheumatism and arthritis:

. . . more of an ossification than is *normal* in body. Hence the
conditions where, with tissue that builds for cartilaginous forces,
becomes centralized, and stiffness ensues, or . . . the flexors of the
muscular forces of forearm become *stiffened* in their activity. 51-1

Regardless of how rheumatism and neuritis had come to develop in
those seeking Cayce's help, his treatments are remarkably consistent.
The same is true of their purpose, which is always to correct underlying
imbalances and reverse the escalation of symptoms. Treatment plans
outlined for almost two thirds of these individuals focus primarily on
dietary advice, tissue manipulation by means of spinal adjustments or
massage, and some form of internal cleansing with electrotherapy running a close fourth.

Dietary corrections are of vital importance in cases of this type, which
involve chemical imbalance. Highly acidic foods, which cause fermentation, and those which lead to extra production of uric acid, such as
certain kinds of meat, seem to create a climate in the digestive system
that is favorable to the development of rheumatic symptoms. Cayce
even goes so far as to say that they would never arise in a sufficiently
alkaline system:

Few germ formations, or none, that injure or cause distress in the
form of neurotic, neuritis or arthritic conditions, or any form of
skin eruption, may come when a system is tended toward
alkalinity!   306-3

Although specifics vary, the following dietary distillation is typical: Eat little or no meat, at least until symptoms ease, concentrating instead on raw and cooked vegetables grown above the ground. Fruit, whole grain cooked cereals, nuts, and the lighter proteins such as eggs and dairy products are beneficial in moderate amounts. Include large amounts of water, always between meals, and go easy on stimulants such as coffee, tea, alcohol, and sugar:

> Do not eat meat other than that of mutton, or goat, or kid. This may be taken in *small* quantities. No other meat or flesh would we take. Let the diet be more of vegetables that grow *above* the ground. None that grow below the ground. Fruits—all of these may be taken in moderation. Drink *plenty* of water. Make it obligatory for self to see that at least two to three *glasses* of water are drunk between each meal—not *at* meals. Not much coffee or tea. Milk may be taken in moderation. *Coffee* not more than once each day.
>
> 92-1

> In the diet, beware of meats—especially of red {raw} meats. Those of the vegetable—those of even more starches—may be better taken than too much of that, that must form acid—and which produce pressure.
>
> 99-5

The goals of spinal adjustments and massage are several: to correct spinal misalignments, reduce undue pressure on nerves and organs, relax tense muscles, and support the flow of blood and lymphatic fluids in their removal of waste products and toxins from the system. This was the purpose of a salt–and–vinegar massage for a fifty–one–year–old woman who was recovering from a fractured wrist:

> . . . we will find this will be a much *better* manner of *relieving* the conditions than by operative measures; for with the massage, not *only* is each bone, or each segment put in its proper position one with another, but their *relations,* of the cushions, or of the cartilage lying between each, are magnified or retarded; that is, built up or removed from, in such a manner as to bring the better activity for the body.
>
> 51-1

Spinal massages with olive oil and myrrh coupled with hot packs of dry salt were advised for a twenty-one-year-old woman suffering from both rheumatism and sciatica, who was assured that: " . . . This, as we see, will soon alleviate the condition." (136-22)

A series of osteopathic adjustments was advised for a woman with rheumatic tendencies:

Q. Is the stiffness in neck due to rheumatism?
A. Due preferably as we find to the specific areas from which infectious forces arise . . . With the adjustments and the stimulations in the areas indicated, these should disappear.   494-2

A careful attentiveness to increasing the body's elimination processes, through methods such as enemas, colonics, herbal tonics, and mild laxatives, will help to relieve toxic buildup and facilitate the release of crystallized elements from afflicted areas. A fifty-six-year-old man who asked about relieving the rheumatism in his right knee was told that this would require: " . . . Relieving the poison from the system." (19-1) A series of colonic irrigations of the large intestine was among the treatments advised.

Internal cleansing through diet and hydration was the main treatment recommended for a twenty-one-year-old woman who asked about alleviating stiffness in both her knees:

Create the proper elimination, and poisons as are gathered by improper circulation will be taken away . . . When we have the full blood supply running through the system, it will take out all drosses . . .   121-1

In a reading given for a forty-two-year-old man, the following exchange took place:

Q. Will the hip and foot continue to improve with present treatment?
A. Continue to improve, so long as the eliminations are kept so that there is not acid reactions, nor the tendency of pressures in

the circulatory forces of the intestinal tract . . .   261-2

Electrotherapy in various forms is advised primarily for its circulation stimulating properties. The following recommendation was made
to a sixty-eight-year-old man who was recovering from lead poisoning:

> For those tendencies of the . . . rheumatic condition, it would be
> well that the . . . violet ray be applied to the superficial portions of
> the body, or that there be the charging of the body throughout with
> same, so as to reduce the salts and allow the eliminations to be
> carried from the system.   287-11

As mentioned earlier, hydrotherapy offers some helpful ways of easing discomfort and stepping up elimination through the pores of the
skin. Dry packs of heated salt, wet Epsom salts poultices, and hot baths
containing large amounts of Epsom salts are most often advised for
these purposes. A thirty-four-year-old woman with rheumatic tendencies in several parts of her body was warned against discontinuing these
baths too soon:

> Leave these off a while, or allow these accumulations, and you'll
> find *rheumatism* will be the natural result; but these are going to
> be eliminated, as the changes come about.   272-6

A constructive attitude of this type is always desirable and will actually make the healing that is needed more likely to occur. Very often
this includes a conscious abstention from negative thoughts:

> Keep *mentally* in that attitude of *constructive* thinking, ever. Never
> allow self to become pessimistic or doubtful, or fearful as to the
> activities about the body in any form.   494-2

In view of the seriousness of some of these conditions, it may be
surprising that Cayce would be so optimistic of success. However, this
was usually the case, provided there was a willingness to complete a
treatment program that might be drawn out over several months. This

proved especially worthwhile in cases where a series of readings took place. One example is the relief of rheumatism in a formerly fractured hip belonging to case 409, a young woman who consulted Cayce several times between the ages of nineteen and twenty-seven. After her first few readings, which recommended a combination of massage, electrotherapy, and elimination aids, the rheumatism was pronounced as cured although her doctors had been highly pessimistic. Now that's inspiring!

Damage Control for Cold Sores and Shingles

For most human gastrointestinal tracts, the annual mega-holiday season that unrolls from Thanksgiving through the start of the New Year is a time of exceptional stress. No, it doesn't require a party to put our long-suffering guts on red alert, but it helps! When the system is chronically overtaxed by sweets, treats, and adult beverages, the distress may be more than just temporary as well. We then risk an increased vulnerability to all types of infectious organisms. Among these, according to the readings, are the herpes viruses that cause cold or canker sores (*simplex*) and shingles (*zoster*). Although this is a smallish topic, Cayce's comments on the eleven or twelve cases of each type are well worth studying.

Herpes simplex is a recurrent viral infection characterized by small, irritating blisters with slightly raised inflammatory bases. This virus takes two forms. HSV-1, the type that commonly causes mouth sores, can also appear on the skin or mucous membranes anywhere in the body, including the eyes. HSV-2 usually affects the genitals. The HSV-1 virus remains sneakily dormant in the nerve ganglia until it is triggered by factors that may be extremely hard to trace. Sun exposure, fever, stress, dietary factors, medications, and suppression of the immune system are all possible culprits.

Herpes zoster may sometimes be confused with herpes simplex, but it rarely recurs and its symptoms are more severe. These larger groups of lesions pop up along the routes of peripheral sensory nerves and can be acutely sensitive to touch. Shingles are activated by the varicella-zoster virus, the same one that causes chicken pox, though they usually appear when childhood bouts are a distant memory. Actually, they can return with a vengeance at any age, but those over fifty are much more vulnerable. Shingles outbreaks may be preceded by uncomfortable sensations that begin in the thoracic regain and generally affect only one side of the body. Blisters on the face can involve an eye to a point requiring professional care. In general, however, there is little that medicine can offer beyond soothing compresses, analgesics, and perhaps antiviral medication. Victims find comfort in the fervent hope that they will never have to go through this again!

Discussions of these two types of herpes in the readings share many common traits. Most are traced, in one way or another, to imbalances involving the body's waste removal system. Indigestion, super-acidity, and poor assimilation of nutrients from foods are typical elements in this toxic cycle. Impaired circulation and general weakness complete the picture of a body under stress. The stage could hardly be more set for a virus that's already lodged in the nervous system.

Here is how Cayce described these developments in several cases of cold sores. Note the mention of acidity in all three and the close connection between acidity and colds in the third:

The disturbances are indicated in the conditions on face, and especially lips, as the result of the great amount of acidity in the system and the . . . necessity . . . for greater eliminations through alimentary canal. 5152-1

. . . the disturbances in the liver *and* the acidity cause the nervous strain through the digestive system, that finds expression at times in the salivary glands in the mouth—soreness, or the irritation on the inside of the mouth and the gums . . . 2771-2

. . . in the present we have a great deal of acidity, which naturally tends to cause the constant contracting of cold. That makes crosses, and that which of course submerges the activities or the coordinating between the circulations through the liver, the kidneys and lungs. These naturally cause a rash, or sores in portions of the body. 2289-6

Similar factors compounded by low energy are clearly at work in the development of shingles. In one case, stress, digestive disturbances, and acidity had affected the capillary circulation, producing " . . . the abrasions as shown in system, causing soreness, tenderness, depression, in the functioning of the organs of elimination." (106-4) Other readings, such as the following, give a more detailed understanding of how lymphatic overloads might occur:

> As to the condition as was given, this was a form of toxin, poison, in system taken into the blood supply and attempting to be eliminated through the capillary circulation . . . *[in]* the lymphatic glands in the cuticle . . . The same we find in the disturbance in the extremities, in the shoulder, arm and in limb, is the deeper accentuation of same condition producing the tenderness, the pain in nerve centers, in the ends of tendons and in muscular forces by toxins in lymphatic, which produce inflammation to these centers, causing distress in the body. The acids as were taken instead of alkalines as given, to produce eliminations, accentuate conditions when the system in its cycle is overtaxed, and we have the results as is seen in body at present.   106-5

In another case, internal cleansing efforts had been complicated by poor food choices:

> As we find, there has been with this body a disregard of those things that were to be the diet for the body. And with the stirring up of the system for proper eliminations there are indications of this in those effects that have been created.   527-3

Still another outbreak of shingles, here on the left side of the face, was attributed to a need for "ionization" (perhaps iron?) as well as to sluggish eliminations:

> As we find, the general weaknesses—and the more specific disturbances which affect the circulatory forces—are the lack of ionization, and hindered eliminations . . . These are indicated in the

> conditions which exist in the circulatory forces in the vegetative
> nerve system especially—and thus the conditions in the face, the
> neck, the arms, the general twitching . . .   2088-1

The symptoms that manifested in these individuals were often acute and quite painful. The cold sores sometimes extended beyond the lips and mouth and in one case were compounded by facial neuralgia. The blisters caused by shingles were especially tender and again involved facial neuralgia in one case. Even their aftereffects, which in some cases had lingered for many months, could be extremely irritating. The readings, however, were always optimistic that correcting core imbalances would bring welcome relief.

Treatments in all of these cases support the body's attempts to strengthen, heal, and, where applicable, prevent further outbreaks. Very broadly, they focus on four areas: relieving discomfort, gently increasing the eliminations, restoring acid–alkaline balance, and stimulating sluggish circulation.

Topical treatments found in cases of cold sores are soothing, alkalizing, and sometimes antiseptic. A lip balm called Camphorice with camphor and mutton tallow as ingredients appears in a few readings, as does a weakened Atomidine solution. The case of neuralgia is addressed with stronger measures, including laudanum and aconite application, warm Epsom salts compresses, and massage with a combination of camphor spirits, turpentine spirits, and mutton tallow. Rinsing the mouth with Glyco-Thymoline or Lavoris can also be advisable:

> Wash or rinse the mouth with Lavoris, full strength. It doesn't hurt
> if a tiny bit is swallowed. Gargle the throat and rinse the mouth
> with this.   3335-1

A favored topical dusting for shingles is a soothing body powder containing stearate of zinc and Peruvian balsam. A somewhat different tack is taken with a combination of sassafras, laudanum, camphor, and glycerin:

> Also, to rid the body of the abrasions or the rash, or the prickly

pin-stabbing pains over portions of the system, around the abdomen and the like, we would prepare a solution to be applied externally, as this . . .   322-5

The types of elimination aids prescribed seem to vary more with the
individual than with the type of herpes involved. External measures
include high enemas, colonics, and abdominal Glyco-Thymoline or castor oil packs. The internal ones, many of which are also digestive aids,
include Al-Caroid; a mixture of sulfur, cream of tartar, and Rochelle
salts; Citrocarbonate, Milk of Magnesia, Milk of Bismuth, Castoria, and
kidney stimulants, such as watermelon seed tea and sweet spirits of nitre.
Short term boosts to normal elimination and digestive functions such
as these are intended to step up the removal of toxins from the intestinal system and circulation while at the same time preventing further
production. Readings given in two cases of shingles comment:

We would follow then closer those suggestions as were given, to
produce the eliminations in the system, to cause the centers in the
intestinal system, in liver, in kidneys, to function through their
normal channels, preventing toxins from being taken into circulation and causing disturbances we find at the present time. 106-5

These will get rid of the conditions of the rash or hives, which has
been indicated on portions of the body, around the abdomen, at a
portion of the side and back . . .   338-9

Dietary directions are given with essentially the same goals, as poor
food choices can be a large part of the problem. Here, the main objec-
tives are raising fiber content, increasing alkalinity, improving nutrition, and avoiding further stress on an already overtaxed digestive
system. To give these functions a break, some menu plans are extremely
light and semiliquid, while others consist mostly of raw vegetables
served grated or ground with oil or dressing, along with moderate
amounts of whole grain cereals, fruit juices, and perhaps light proteins.
Warnings target foods that are highly acidic, hard on the digestive system, or lacking in nutritional value, such as sugar, refined starches, vin-

egar, and anything fried. Since vegetables and fruits (though apples are sometimes banned) are generally alkaline forming, they are definitely what Cayce has in mind:

> Do that, and only needs the body rest from foods for system, save those of the nature that reduces the acid, the repelling force in the emunctories, and allow the system to come to its normal condition.
> 106-4

> . . . in the diet use more fresh, raw vegetables, especially do have more watercress and all forms of foods which are grated or ground but do prepare them with the juices.
> 338-9

Restoration of acid–alkaline balance is typically accomplished through diet and elimination aids such as those already mentioned. However, severe problems with acidity might also warrant some tiny doses of Glyco-Thymoline in water. The prescription given in two cases of cold sores was two to five drops in a glass of water taken two or three times a day. Local applications and gargles, as found in other readings and a few later reports, would, of course, have a similar effect.

Cayce's usual methods of boosting sluggish circulation in these cases are massage, other forms of hydrotherapy such as sweats, and spinal manipulation when needed. One treatment in a case of cold sores complicated by neuralgia is osteopathic massage from the head and neck downward to set up drainages for better eliminations. Spinal adjustments are advised to remove the stress on nerve centers in another case of cold sores, and regular massages in a third. Similarly, upper spine adjustments are prescribed in one case of shingles and massage in another:

> Also each day we should have a gentle massage, especially through the areas between the shoulders—from the waist to the base of the brain, but particularly between the shoulders—with an equal combination of Peanut Oil and Olive Oil. This as we find will make for a better stimulation.
> 2088-1

> These will be materially aided by the massages setting up better

eliminations, or coordination between the alimentary canal and
the general superficial circulation.   3335-1

Electrotherapy would be advised for similar purposes. The above
reading also proposed the following classic Cayce aid to meditation,
circulation balance, and restful sleep:

> Use also the Radio-Active Appliance as an equalizer and as an aid
> to re-ionization of the circulation, and as an aid to rest and quiet.
>   2088-1

The need for rest and quiet does seem especially important in cases
of shingles, perhaps because of the close connection between emotions,
the nervous systems, and the circulation:

> If there are the worries and aggravations, these worries and ag-
> gravations will reflect in the functioning of the organs of the cen-
> tral nerve and blood supply as well as in the sympathetic. 338-9

Cayce's frequent advice to maintain a positive attitude reflects his
general optimism about eliminating even long–standing symptoms of
both cold sores and shingles from the system. The course of improvement can be slow, however, as those with shingles can attest. Even cold
sores can take some time to reverse when they are persistent and severe, as was the case with a man whose treatment cycle was projected
to take six to eight weeks. The results, however, are bound to be worth
all the effort:

> And at the end of three such rounds we find that these tenden-
> cies—for the soreness, the breaking out, for cold, all of these con-
> ditions—will be *gone!*   779-21

Hope for Hives

Most people experience hives, or urticaria, as an eruptive skin response to an irritant to which the body has been exposed. These irritat-

ing pustules in the dermal layer of the akin are basically anaphylactic in nature, though they're limited to the skin and the tissues beneath it. They may even look and feel like the results of a nasty bee encounter, giving a possible clue to the descriptive origin of the word hives. A long list of possible irritants includes medications, insect bites and stings, desensitization injections, certain foods (such as shellfish, eggs, nuts, fruit, or alcohol), sunlight, heat, cold, and mild trauma. However, the culprit is not always known, and hives lasting longer than three weeks are especially hard to deal with. Oral antihistamines usually relieve the symptoms but not the underlying cause.

Commentaries on these pesky outbreaks can be found in eighteen readings given for fifteen individuals who ranged widely in age. Some of these conditions were extremely longstanding. The record was held by a thirty-nine-year-old woman who had reportedly suffered from hives for three years!

Not surprisingly, Cayce's comments on the origins of these outbreaks have much in common with those made in cases of shingles and other types of skin disturbances. Super acidity, toxins in the bloodstream, sluggish elimination, poor circulation, liver-kidney imbalances, congestion, and emotional aggravation are all often cited factors. Found in any combination, they interfere with the ability to process any additional stressor that impacts the lymphatic system:

> As we find, there are still some disturbances through the soft tissue of face, nasal passages, antrums and the like. These, with a toxic condition that arises from a super-acidity in the bloodstream, and with a congestion in same through the abdominal area, tend to produce poisons in the system that are irritating . . .
> Q. Why the hives?
> A. Poor circulation . . .   257-208

> The reaction caused from this in the present is a hindrance to the circulation to the lower extremities . . . from the lack of proper eliminations, from the uric acids and the tendency for an excess acidity throughout the system; a rash, or what might be called the hives or the like, about portions of the abdomen and chest.   2534-1

Q. What causes breaking out with hives or itching bumps?
A. Poisons from system, as we have indicated.   356-2

The body is susceptible to conditions that come or affect the body
from without, through the sympathetic system, as well as through
those of the distributions in the eliminating system; so that we
have such hindrances as is manifested in the eliminations, especially as seen in the skin, or an irritation as of a rash—as between
fingers, feet or in portions where the lymph or emunctory circulation is nearest the skin . . .   1734-4

Thus the form of irritation in the lymph circulation attempting to
eliminate the poisons that should be carried through the drosses
of the body.   3201-1

Q. What is the physical explanation of hives, and how may I overcome this condition?
A. These are from lack of proper eliminations and of allowing self
to become aggravated and breaking the connections between
cerebrospinal and sympathetic nervous systems . . . for these destructive attitudes bring on self all the pent up feelings and they
find expression in irritations.   5226-1

The above excerpts describe factors and states of imbalance that pre-
dispose the body to allergic reaction. Although specific triggers of hives
vary in these cases, most seem to be of dietary origin. An exception is a
reaction to gold salts, a medication prescribed in a case of arthritis. An
allergy to beer and high alcohol beverages is the subject of emphatic
warnings in another case:

Light wines may be taken, but not strong drinks nor any fermentations as of beer or hops—for these are not well—the body is allergic to these.   257-208

Other readings warn against acid–forming foods in general, at least
for the time being:

Q. Are there any specific things to which he is allergic?
A. As long as there is kept too much acid in the system, or those foods or combinations that produce acid, he will be allergic—of course—to these things that are in the nature tending to make this acidity.   3201-1

A reaction to legumes is the culprit in a more unusual case:

Q. What type of foods or articles of food seem to be persistently causing the hives?
A. Those of any nature as from any form of dried beans or the like. The body is allergic to these; dried peas, beans or such.   2534-2

Which foods, besides the above, qualify as acid producing? These readings advise against items such as white bread, sugar, meat fats, fried foods, and in a couple of cases, white potatoes and shellfish. Some also target over eating and poor food combining as factors in acidity and indigestion.

Treatment recommendations for hives focus mostly on stepping up eliminations, improving acid–alkaline balance, stimulating the circulation, correcting any spinal pressures, and reducing congestion where applicable. A diet that helps the body cleanse, balance, and strengthen is clearly a major form of treatment here.

A therapeutic diet is light, easily digested, and perhaps even semiliquid for those under severe gastric stress. Aiding both eliminations and alkalinity naturally requires a super abundance of fresh vegetables, especially when they're raw, green, and leafy. Watercress and other salad vegetables are best grated or ground and served with their own juices. Other foods to emphasize include soups, cooked vegetables, and fruit. Whole grain cereals, eggs, dark bread, the lighter meats, and unrefined sweets provide some needed balance. Using only sea or kelp salt is occasionally mentioned. Drinking plenty of water is always optimal.

Additional measures may well be needed to speed the elimination of toxins and normalize the state of the intestines. First among these are colonics and enemas:

These will get rid of the conditions of the rash or hives, which has
been indicated on portions of the body, around the abdomen, at a
portion of the side and back . . .   338-9

Laxatives may also be in order with the readings favoring those that
are also soothing to the digestive tract, such as Milk of Magnesia, Milk
of Bismuth, Castoria, Sal Hepatica, and Eno salts. Or, perhaps, a castor
oil pack series that concludes with a dose of olive oil is most
appropriate.

Hydrotherapy is a pleasant way to help the pores of the skin throw
off toxins and to stimulate general circulation. Cayce's methods include
fume baths with witch hazel, needle showers, and Epsom salts baths.
Treatments typically end with a soothing rubdown using peanut oil or
pine oil. Or, the electric vibrator massage found in one case could be a
stimulating alternative.

Spinal adjustments fine-tune the circulation and may at the same
time aid the digestion by balancing nerve impulses to various parts of
the body. In the readings, " . . . the osteopathic corrections are for the
general condition and to correct the causes, while the hydrotherapy is
for the acute condition of the hives or to eliminate the poisons from the
system." (3201-1) Exercise, when the body can handle it, is an ideal addition.

Topical applications in these cases are rare. One reading mentions a
product known as D.D.D. Liquid. (257-208) Another gives antiseptic instructions:

And where there is the rash—or the indication of the lack of proper
eliminations—bathe the body in a very weakened antiseptic solution. Or, to a pint of water put at least ten drops of a good strong
antiseptic. This may be of any nature—preferably that of an
alkalin-reacting nature; as Lavoris or Glyco-Thymoline.   2102-1

Some readings made optimistic remarks about the results of the suggested treatments. Of the few reports that were received, one case of
giant hives was pronounced as cured, though other respondents, while
delighted about improvements in overall health, were still waiting for

the skin eruptions to disappear.

Yes, there is hope for hives, but results can slow in coming. In the mean time, it's best to focus on internal cleansing and avoid doing anything rash!

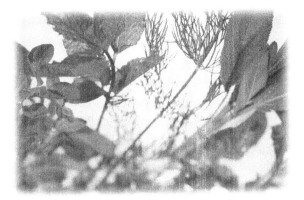

Holistic Perspectives

Healing Rocks

Most, if not all, of us find ourselves drawn to the mineral world in some way. This attraction may take very specific forms, such as lapis earrings, an amethyst pendant, a gold watch, or a ruby ring. Some of us have even wondered why we favor certain stones. Is it their color, value, or a more elusive factor such as how they make us feel?

The lore of ancient cultures reveals a highly developed system of usage for precious and semiprecious stones. Amulets were worn for protection, charms for luck, tokens for love, and talismans as reminders of a noble goal. Therapeutic uses, which were extremely varied, ranged from antidotes for alcoholism and insomnia to salves for wounds. Psychic stones were used to invite dreams, visions, and the opening of the third eye. A link with astrology gave rise to birthstones—a popularized fragment of this esoteric science.

The Edgar Cayce readings agree that the vibrations of the right gems, stones, and metals can be extremely helpful and supportive influences. They also note that individual responses to the same minerals, colors, and designs will vary, due to multiple factors that include past life associations. With this in mind, here are some of Cayce's fascinating comments on the healing uses of these treasures from the earth (except for lapis, which deserves its own in depth study).

The **pearl**, which has always been treasured, is regarded as a positive influence in twelve readings. Wearing or keeping it close comes advised for a variety of purposes, including healing, creativity, purity, strength, peace, and keeping an even temperament. Other helpful stones sometimes associated with the pearl are moonstone, ruby, bloodstone, opal, and jade. The origin of this lustrous stone is regarded as part of its effect on the wearer: "The pearl should be worn upon the body, or against the flesh . . . for its vibrations are healing as well as creative—because of the very irritation as produced same . . . " (951-4)

The **ruby**, one of the most highly valued gemstones, is recommended just as often. In the readings it is regarded as an aid to mental concentration, a source of strength, a creative stimulant, and an incentive in focusing on the spiritual side of life. Associated stones include bloodstone, onyx, pearl, moonstone, and chalcedony. Regarding the power of this gem to amplify constructive thoughts, Cayce notes: ". . . if the ruby is kept close to the body, it will bring strength, power and might . . . to the purposes set by the entity, or those choices given." (2571-1)

The **bloodstone**, suggested in ten readings, also imparts the vitality of the color red with a background of grounding green. It is sometimes recommended in combination with, or as an alternative to, ruby, lapis lazuli, moonstone, and pearl. Due to ". . . the emanations from high electrical forces from its copper base" (816-3), this mineral has a healing, strengthening, creative, and calming influence: " . . . There are those to whom the bloodstone brings harmony, and less of the tendencies for anger . . . " (5294-1)

The milky, glowing **moonstone** is recommended in nine readings for its strengthening, uplifting, and protective properties, and is associated at times with bloodstone, pearl, and agate. Remarking that some moonstone wearers ". . . might find that it would bring peace, harmony and those tendencies towards spiritual things" (5294-1), Cayce told one individual that: " . . . It will give strength, and it will keep that which is nearest to you closer to you; not as an omen but as a part of your mental and spiritual consciousness." (5125-1)

The **amethyst**, which can be found in six cases, is a form of clear, crystalline quartz that has been valued as a healing and attunement aid since ancient times. Similar properties, along with temper control in one case, are found in the readings. This gemstone is sometimes to be used with chrysolite, ivory, and agate. As an aid in quieting the mind, the vibration of amethyst is found to " . . . bring greater harmony, in not only body but in the mental attributes." (1986-1)

Coral, advised in the same number of cases, was once highly prized as a protective charm. The readings regard it as a soothing aid to attunement with the Creative Forces and the vibrations of water. One individual was told that: " . . . Coral should be about the entity at all times; worn—not as a charm, {but for} the vibrations of the body as related to same. Because of the very nature of its construction, and the very activity of the soul forces . . . this would become a helpful influence . . . " (2073-2)

The **opal**, with its rainbow play of colors, is mentioned with the same frequency. Once regarded as one of the most powerful healing stones in the world, this scintillating amalgam of quartz and water is definitely considered intense by Cayce. Often associated with moonstone, the opal is regarded as a bringer of passion that can be spiritually directed: ". . . the fire opal would be of the stones that should be about the entity; for the holding of that fire, that vigor, that *understanding* that makes for purification . . . " (1193-1)

Several additional stones mentioned only a few times are notable for Cayce's intriguing comments. Here are a few examples:

Hence we find the agate, the beryl, should be *stones* with the vibrations and under the influence that the entity may find carrying an incense to the finer self that makes for an awakening, an opening of the inner self for the *receptiveness.*   707-1

We find that the crystal as a stone, or any white stone, has a helpful influence—if carried about the body . . .   2285-1

We find jade as combined with pearls unusual in their effect upon the entity, especially in moods . . . These would be helpful, then . . . when seeking to give expression of that which is either felt in the emotional self or for the accomplishing of same.   1189-1

Ye should find the diamond and the ruby close to your body oft, for their vibrations will keep the vibrations of the body in better attune with infinity and not with purely mental or material things of life.   5322-1

. . . keep the topaz as a stone about thee always. Its beauty, its purity, its clarity, may bring to thee strength.   2281-1

Comments, such as the above, inspire one to experiment or perhaps to seek out a reading on the subject. Equipped with an open mind, you'll never meet a rock you dislike.

The Case of the Elusive Singing Lapis

Of all the potentially confusing bodies of commentary in the Cayce readings, there are few that compare in head-scratching potential with those made about "lapis." Since few stones are also so glowingly recommended, many have bent their intelligence to the task of solving this little mystery. Those who wish to play detective themselves will appreciate a sketch of the facts.

In the world of semiprecious stones, there are at least three kinds of lapis. Any of the following may or may not be the objects of our quest.

Lapis lazuli, regarded by ancient alchemists as the stone of heaven, is noted for its many rich shades of blue, often accompanied by a grayish matrix and tiny flecks of pyrite. Few stones have been more highly valued, especially by the mystically oriented cultures of ancient Egypt and China.

Lapis linguis occurs in various shades of blue as well, as its other name, **azurite**, denotes. Found in the upper oxidized portions of copper deposits, it is usually linked with malachite. Azurite was reportedly considered a stone of great power in ancient Egypt, where it was used for spiritual guidance, clairvoyance, and healing.

Lapis ligurius, or **malachite**, is a green, often banded, copper ore that derives its name from the Greek word for mallow, a plant with bright green leaves. Malachite has been a favorite since ancient times for its protective, healing, and cosmetic uses.

There are close to thirty Cayce references, by name, to these types of lapis, making it the most recommended general category of stone in the readings.

Lapis lazuli is especially valued for its strengthening, healing, and spiritualizing influences, as the following comments show:

> Keep something blue, and especially the color and emanations of the lapis lazuli; not the slick or polished nature, but of that nature that the emanations from same may give life and vitality. 2132-1

> Upon thy body wear the lapis lazuli, which bringeth strength to thy weakened and faltering body at times. The vibrations . . . may again bring in thy consciousness the awareness that life itself, health itself, cometh from the Creator.   2564-3

> So may . . . those vibrations . . . with metals such as come in the lapis lazuli, make for the raising of the attunement in self through meditation.   707-1

> This if encased and worn upon the breast would bring healing, and decisions for the entity, because of the very vibrations that such create in their activity.   2282-1

Several readings, as in the one just quoted, suggest that the lapis be enclosed in a transparent substance such as crystal or glass. Apparently this has the effect of making the vibrations less intense:

> As to stones—have near to self, wear preferably upon the body, about the neck, the lapis lazuli; this preferably encased in crystal. It will be not merely as an ornament but as strength from the emanation which will be gained by the body always from same.
>   1981-1

> The lapis lazuli would be very good for the body, if it were worn in

crystal next to the skin.   2376-1

Lapis linguis, . . . lapis lazuli. This as we find might be said to be a part of that same composition referred to; for it carries that vibration which will give strength to the body. Well that this be preserved between thin layers of glass or such compositions, else its radiation is too great.   1931-2

Much like lapis lazuli, lapis linguis is said by Cayce to promote mental clarity, deeper meditations, and even the development of psychic abilities. It seems no coincidence that the name is a Latin term meaning "speaking stone:"

Of particular value to those who are interested in things psychic! {It will} . . . aid an individual in its contact with the higher sources of activity!   440-2

. . . those that are of a psychic turn may hear . . . those vibrations giving off, or the singing or talking stones—as they have been called in places.   440-11

. . . the lapis linguis also would bring to the entity much, if it were worn about the body, keeping low the fires of passion—from materiality that there may be greater mental and spiritual development of this entity in the experience.   559-7

Hence, as we find the wearing of the stone lapis linguis would be as an aid in its meditative periods, and would become as a helpful influence.   1058-1

Although the blue tones seem vastly favored, green lapis ligurius is also sometimes suggested for properties such as healing and protection:

Not that these should be merely considered as good luck stones that the entity should wear about self often, or most always—but the lapis ligurius . . . would bring much that will act in that manner as would be termed a *protective* influence . . . This is the green stone, you see—the crystallization of copper and those influences that are creative within themselves.   1931-1

The lapis lazuli, worn close to the body would be well for the general health . . . *{It's}* an erosion *{corrosion}* of copper, but this encased in a glass . . . would be well. The color is green. Hence the entity should ever be as a healing influence to others . . . 3416-1

Wait a moment—lapis lazuli, *green?* Are we scratching our heads yet? Consider the readings that refer to lazuli, linguis, and copper as though they are all describing the same stone—perplexing because lapis lazuli is not a copper derivative:

For the entity should ever wear about the body the lapis lazuli or the lapis linguis; for these will bring strength to the body . . .
                                                                        691-1

The lapis lazuli stone would be well to wear about the body. This is as a chrysalis to be sure of copper; thus the very natures of same produce those emanations . . . in which the environ is made for keeping holy things holy, and material things in their proper relationships. For it acts as it were as a storage of energies for the inner self.   880-2

We find that it would be very helpful for the entity to wear upon the body a piece of stone that is of the lapis lazuli variety, but the essence or fusion of copper; not as a charm but as a helpful force in the vibrations that will coordinate with the body.   1651-2

To compound the confusion just a tad further, several readings suggest locating a huge specimen of lapis in the New York Museum of Natural History in order to listen to it "sing." Here, Cayce asserts that the composition of this stone is ". . . Not lapis linguis, but *lapis!*" (440-9) Strangely, all other readings in this series refer specifically to lapis linguis or azurite.

So, what's an investigator to do with all these discrepancies? When faced with terminology problems of this magnitude, could it be that it's time to rethink the terms themselves? In that case, the problem becomes basically one of associating a mineral description with the proper name. We're looking for a copper derivative that is soft blue, or occasionally green in color, related to lapis linguis and ligurius, and found in Arizona.

The stone that actually matches all these characteristics is chrysocolla, a more rare form of copper with the brilliant blues and aquas of a tropical shore. Chrysocolla is definitely a stone that sings.

Of course there's no way to prove in a court of law that this is what the readings had in mind or in what percentage of cases. It's entirely possible that in some instances, lapis lazuli or azurite is exactly what is meant. But there are two things we know for sure, beyond any shadow of a doubt: Cayce's source can be extremely literal at times, and both names have the same meaning: "blue stone."

Essential Oils: More than Just a Pretty Fragrance

As all can see on the labels of common household products, the notion of feel-good aromas has become a major commercial ploy. Consider the anti-stress aromatherapy dish soap with lavender and ylang-ylang essences that promises to turn a chore into a soothing and unwinding experience. The rich violet-colored liquid and bottle top are extra cues to the novel concept of work as pleasure.

Well, these promoters have done their research. Lavender, one of the most universally positive aromas, is generally regarded as calming and balancing, while relaxing ylang-ylang is said to have sensual and even euphoric overtones. Hmmm—dishes for two, anyone?

But wait—better check the label before getting too excited. Real aromatherapy benefits require genuine essential oils.

These volatile, highly concentrated essences are derived from leaves, blossoms, stems, fruit, or roots, usually by steam or water distillation. Sometimes known as "plant hormones," they embody the unique flavors, aromas, and energy patterns of growing things. When microparticles of essential oils are released into the air or absorbed by the skin, our odor receptors send signals directly to the brain, activating hormonal and even chemical changes. With the right aromas, we literally begin to feel better.

Practitioners of aromatherapy claim that the transformative potential of plant essences lies in their power to evoke our deepest memories and emotions. Some readings acknowledge this, although most focus on physical, rather than psychological, therapies. Following are some prime examples:

Cedarwood

Aromatic, woodsy-smelling *Juniperus virginiana* is probably most often associated with pencil shavings and gerbil cages. However, the oil of this US plant is traditionally used as a general tonic, sensual stimulant, inhalant ingredient, and insect repellant. Cedarwood can also be helpful for troubled skin and hair. Recommended by Cayce in massage, its applications include bath oil, facial wash, inhalant ingredient, and closet scent. Avoid during pregnancy.

Eucalyptus

The strong, clean-smelling extract of *Eucalyptus globulus*, from the fresh leaves of Australian and Chinese trees, is probably the best-known pure essential oil and is a medicine cabinet staple. A common Cayce inhalant ingredient, eucalyptus is used to clear the chest and sinuses and ease breathing. It also makes a fresh addition to household cleaning products and even repels insects. A couple of drops will do the job when adding to bath water, air fresheners, facial steams, or massage formulas. Avoid with homeopathic remedies.

Fir Needle

Just a few drops of this rich, piney oil are enough to release the festive aroma of a whole roomful of Christmas trees! The fragrant essence of Canadian *Abies alba* is another Cayce inhalant ingredient used to open breathing passages and tone the respiratory system. Add to bath water or massage oils for muscle and joint relief or mist into the air for an effect that is soothing and revitalizing at the same time.

Lavender

Lavandula officinalis, an aromatherapy classic often derived from French flowers, is a relaxing and especially balancing scent with many applications. Derived from the Latin *lavāre*, that means "to wash," the name reflects centuries of use as a purifying herb. Lavender has numerous uses in skin care, inhalation, stress reduction, and much more. It makes a soothing addition to body oils and skin care preparations and has been misted into the air of British hospitals to help patients sleep. According to Cayce, the scent can even be used as a meditation aid!

Pine Needle

The natural essence of *Pinus pumilio* captures all the invigorating, decongestant properties of a walk in a pine forest. The oil derived from its health-giving needles is highly valued as an inhalant by both Cayce and traditional sources. Considered stimulating and warming, it is included in many toiletry and pharmaceutical preparations for its pleasantly clean scent. Pine needle oil is also a favorite household fragrance when added to air fresheners, carpet refreshers, and floor cleaning solutions. It can cause skin irritation, so use with caution.

Sassafras

With a sweet, woodsy fragrance that is linked in memory with root beer and soda fountains, this plant is probably best known for the delicious tea that is brewed from the bark of the root. Known for its warming properties, the presence of sassafras oil in many Cayce massage formulas may aid in stimulating circulation. The aroma of this US plant is pungent and therapeutic.

Wintergreen

More than just a chewing gum and breath mint flavor, this refreshing essence is a key ingredient in some of Cayce's more stimulating massage formulas. When used diluted on the skin, *Gaultheria procumbens* provides soothing relief and increased circulation. Mild chest-clearing properties add to its effectiveness as a bath water addition and inhalant ingredient. Avoid during pregnancy.

The Cayce essential oils make a healthy introduction to the wide world of environmental fragrances. Just remember to start with extremely small amounts, such as one drop on an incense ring or five in the bath. These oils are highly concentrated and must be diluted to avoid burns. Now, it's time to wash some dishes. All this nice purple detergent needs is some real essential oils!

Transforming Stress

It's ridiculously easy to succumb to stress before we even realize what hit us. Physical crises, emotional tension, and economic crunch times all tend to undermine our sense of security in such seemingly logical ways that fear finds a way to slip in. Then, in a true lapse of logic, we forget that pushing the panic button actually impairs our ability to cope. In fact, it is such an effective stress producer in its own right that unpleasant consequences are bound to follow.

This is the gist of the Cayce perspective, which encompasses many words of wisdom on this timely topic. Not the least of these is the observation that "stress" is a word with several different, though closely related, meanings. It connotes not only a perceived negative, as in strain or tension, but also the neutral or positive concept of emphasis. Then there is the closely related "distress," conveying affliction, perplexity, or pain. The presence of all three in some of the same readings suggests a link between the type of stress a person is under and the type of distress that manifests, along with clues to what needs to be stressed at the time.

Examining this information like good detectives yields some valuable life tools not only for relieving unnecessary stress, but also for confronting realities with a more positive, focused response. In order to unravel our own riddles, we must first acknowledge, with Cayce, that life stress, as in potentially tension–producing situations, is universal. The difference lies in how we learn to handle it. The most constructive approach is to treat each stressful event as a test, challenge, growth opportunity, or even a cherished gift. With this kind of attitude we're always prepared to learn something, whether that is temper control, mental skills, or something entirely different:

> It may be said that the experience then was such that the stress and strain made for *mental* development . . .   967-1

> These are inclinations, these may find expressions at times under stress or strain; but used properly, as has been given, may be helpful. For they without a temper are not very worth while, but they with a temper not controlled are worthless.   1244-1

The catch in this approach is, of course, that we are now required to be responsible for our responses, i.e. grow up. If that's easier said than done, then fresh motivation in the form of unpleasant physical symptoms will eventually arise. This, too, is an important learning experience:

> For the mental, we find, were those things and conditions as bring the mental distress laid aside more often, that this would *relieve* the distress, and we would find that the activities in the direction *of* alleviating these worries would be much improved; for the body, as many an individual, should know that the worrying only brings for self detrimental conditions, and very seldom—if ever—aids in meeting conditions better, but rather unfits one for the stress as is brought to bear.   372-2

When this type of distress is in its early stages, a change in attitude coupled with some much needed rest and relaxation may be all that's required to correct it. This was Cayce's advice to an individual who had been "working under heavy strain" and had already had some physical problems:

Rather these precautions should be taken, and we will prevent further disorders and bring about the abilities for the body to function better physically and mentally; for irritations, or weaknesses, or distress, must work to a bad effect upon the abilities and mental efficiencies of the body—or *any* body.   437-6

Other readings offer thoughtful lectures about the health challenges people are inviting in through worry and anxiety:

When there have been periods of adhering to the suggestions indicated, improvements have come. And then because of the apparent stress of circumstance, or the desire to excel in some definite direction, the body has—through associations, or through activities—been prompted to break over from those conditions and those things outlined for the body for the better health.

And *now* the body finds itself anxious about conditions.

If this is allowed to become of such natures as to cause the body to become panicky, or so over anxious as to do those things against which it has been warned, then it will meet the consequences of same.   257-217

For, with the worrying—or anxiety—inner anxiety (for the body is an emotional body), it works on the emotions of the body when there is the indication of suffering of any kind. These all aggravate the disturbances to the body itself. It dims the vision, it cuts the appetite, it makes for overactivity of the kidneys, it destroys the proper circulation through the abdominal area, and the body becomes aware of being very tired, very much worn, and of the aggravations to the organs of the pelvis, the kidney, the bladder and the digestive system throughout.

These, as we find, may be corrected. It will require, of course, one thing—that the body change the general mental attitude.
          3098-1

The role of emotion in physical stress also works in reverse. Medical science agrees with this in principle in attributing emotional instability and hypersensitivity to various physical or "chemical" imbalances. However, the readings tend to see the nature of these imbalances differently, attributing most to a lack of coordination between the cerebrospinal and sympathetic (autonomic) nervous systems, caused by injury or other factors:

> The *nervous system,* through stress and strains, at times has made and does make for too much of the imaginative forces *controlling* the emotional forces in the system, rather than the reasoning through normalcy. Not that these are altogether neurotic conditions, but these tendencies have existed from the very beginnings when there were those reactions that caused or produced these toxic forces in the system that brought about the condition in the area as indicated.   279-20

> Q. How can I improve my powers of concentration?
> A. When there is removed a great deal of that distress between coordinations of the cerebrospinal and sympathetic system, these should come back to near normal reactions—and concentration will be easier for the body.
> Q. What can I do to secure better emotional stability?
> A. This is of the mental self, that—with the correction of the nerve pressures—may be controlled within self.   2771-2

Once the nature of our particular stressors is understood, it's time to begin to correct them. Of course, some types of treatments are almost always helpful, regardless of how the tension or imbalance originated.

Firstly, most readings for the excessively stressed recommend a series of osteopathic adjustments to improve nervous system coordination. Proper alignment of the spinal vertebrae has far-reaching health benefits, including calmer nerves, looser muscles, and improved circulation. Regular massages, to be given along with the adjustments or separately, have many of the same relaxing and balancing effects:

> Yet, we find much relief might be had through the massage of tendons in the right shoulder and in the upper dorsal and cervical

area, and by some alignments in the dorsal and cervical area; for this would relieve a great deal the conditions for the head and the tendency for the direction of the impulses in the sensory system . . .   478-2

How can we know whether our spines are properly aligned? Evidently, one sign of this is an enviable emotional control, as one reading explains:

Hence there is perfect coordination between the sympathetic and cerebrospinal system. So, when the body desires or wishes or feels that it is more to the betterment of conditions or surroundings to be enthusiastic, it can be enthusiastic immediately. If it desires, or it meets the conditions that it be rather submerged and a more general or more specific condition be exercised, the abilities in these directions are to withhold emotion or withhold influences that would exercise through sentiment or the emotional side of the individual entity.   440-2

The importance of elimination aids in stress reduction cannot be overestimated. Gentle laxatives and the occasional enema or colonic clear the system of toxins, which keep it from functioning at its best:

Keep the intestinal tract open, using enemas occasionally to cleanse the colon, for this will reduce the toxic condition in system and, removing the stress, will overcome various conditions . . .
86-1

Exercise, especially when taken outdoors, is an important way to relieve areas of tension on an individually tailored basis:

The exercises would be for that portion of the body that is under stress at each time the body should take the exercise, which is night and morning. At times we will find this shifted from the abdomen to the pelvis, again to the extremities, again to the limbs and shoulders. Each should be exercised in the manner as to give

the release of the tissue and muscular forces of that portion of the
body.   26-1

A diet to prevent or relieve stress should be well balanced and easy
on the sweets, starches, and heavy meats. Drinking plenty of water is
also helpful:

> Of course, as the body has learned, be mindful of not eating heavy
> meats when under stress or strain.   696-2

> Q. Any other suggestions for the relief and improvement of this
> body?
> A. Drink more water.   294-64

General hydrotherapy measures, including sweats, rubdowns, baths,
and needle showers, are often advised for those under stress to stimulate circulation, promote elimination of toxins, and relax the nerves. A
pleasant sleep–inducing massage alternative is an electric vibrator treatment given at bedtime:

> Q. What can be given to help body sleep at night?
> A. The gentle relaxation of the body by the electrical driven stimu-
> lator, or vibrator, will aid in relieving this distress . . . when worry is
> left off.   372-2

Cayce's reminder that the treatment will only work with the right
attitude brings us full circle to the need for some new mental habits.
The above reading advises the discipline of substituting anxiety about
finances with other thoughts along with a sense of trust in a higher
power:

> Q .What relief is there for the mental condition of body regarding
> financial conditions in the present?
> A. Do not worry about these conditions. How to prevent worry?
> Then fill the mind with *other* conditions, knowing that these will
> be—and are being taken care of.   372-2

Other readings recommend improving one's sense of harmony with that higher power and adhering to already existent ideals:

Not that there are not periods when there will not be influences from without as well as from within that will cause emotional or mental and physical reactions that cause an awareness of disturbances, but keeping in attunement and in at-onement with the Creative Influences we become aware of those things necessary.

1158-22

Not that the desire of self would be to induce or impel others to think as self . . . but rather that self . . . lives . . . in its acts, in its words, in its deeds, in keeping with that which it has set as its ideal.   1315-10

Still another valuable practice is to harness a strong imagination by visualizing all physical functions working properly together and the health continuously improving:

Then, as the body knows, that as is to be held before the body as the mental image, is to be seen—the eliminations being carried on properly, the throwing off of those congested forces and eliminations being nominal, these on the improve, these being made well, will make for bettered conditions in the body . . .   264-13

Clearly, there are many helpful ways of transforming a bugaboo that is stressful or causing distress into a life–changing new discovery that is just begging to be stressed. In the absence of certainty, the best place to start is just about anywhere. Take a break, a hike, a sweat, a back crack, a rubdown, a colon cleanse, an ideals workshop, a good meal, an herbal tonic, some calming minerals, a positive thinking exercise, or a sizeable slug of water, keeping in mind the familiar adjunct: Why worry when you can pray?

Allergies: All in the Body-Mind

From hay fever and asthma to eczema and hives, allergic reactions are never pleasant, although they can be many other things, including mild, severe, escalating, exasperating, embarrassing, scary, painful, or even fatal in their extreme. All stem from an enhanced sensitivity to some type of irritant. Contributing factors are so diverse that those who suspect others of overreacting could easily be right, or totally wrong.

Respiratory allergies can be chronic as in some cases of asthma, seasonal like hay fever, or intermittent depending on the amount of dust, smoke, animal dander, or other factors in the environment. The irritants that lead to skin reactions can be of external (contact dermatitis) or internal (food allergies) origin, or sometimes both. All of these can be coped with, but wouldn't it be life changing if they didn't have to be? The Edgar Cayce readings offer that hope.

Then, as now, the precipitating causes of allergies in these readings were all over the map. Offending items included beer, fur, household pets, feathers, odors, dust, flowers, pollen, plants, lint, specific foods, food combinations, tobacco smoke, dye, paint fumes, weather, wool, sprays, chemicals, noises, sunlight, metals, colors, negative vibrations, and even certain suggestions! Today we would add medications, bites, stings, food additives, and environmental toxins.

The first step in treatment remains to remove the irritants from the body's vicinity, or the body from the vicinity if necessary, while symptoms ease. Some of the changes thus entailed might be unwelcome, or even rather drastic. Those who are aggravating their symptoms with the wrong foods, beverages, or harmful combinations need to quit doing so, and stop acting like they are not to blame for their alarming intestinal reactions:

As has been indicated, the body—through the alimentary canal—is allergic to malt; and those foods, and especially of drink, as beer, tend to cause a greater flow of the lymph through those areas when such are taken.   257-204

Children are not exempt from dietary and other restrictions. An allergic youngster who is itching for a feline or canine friend may need to focus on health improvement, starting by laying off the sweets: " . . . Leave off your dogs and cats, and don't eat chocolate." (3053-1)

Environmental exposure is often work related, and a person reacting to irritants (in one case, aluminum dust) may need to change jobs. Advice for those with hay fever will naturally vary with its severity, ranging from a complete change of environment to simply being careful around the garden for a while:

And, in the activities, avoid working with some of the flowers. Avoid any of those that throw off pollen at this particular time.

1541-12

Although avoidance and medication will reliably bring symptomatic relief, they have their limitations. In Cayce's view, allergies are signs of imbalance, and the symptoms are apt to worsen over time. Proper treatment begins with an understanding of how these sensitivities originate, for, as one reading put it: " . . . The pressures come from the external effect, to be sure, but the causes are internal." (3330-1)

A major factor in the development of allergies is an excess of toxins in the intestinal system. This is probably to be expected in cases of food sensitivities:

Q. What can be done to conquer the many allergies to certain fruits and vegetables that I am afflicted with? Is the cause psychological?
A. Cleanse the system! These arise from toxic conditions through the alimentary canal.   3356-2

One contributing factor or even central cause of this toxicity is an overly acidic intestinal system. Acid-forming foods and combinations will put extra strain on an already taxed digestion. The result is a reaction to the offending foods:

Q. Are there any specific things to which he is allergic?

A. As long as there is kept too much acid in the system, or those
foods or combinations that produce acid, he will be allergic—of
course—to those things that are in the nature tending to make this
acidity.   3201-1

An eventual result of intestinal imbalance is the slowing of blood
and lymph circulation. This impairs the body's ability to deal with poor
food choices and other irritants:

Not precautious enough about the diet, and we have again a great
deal of the humor that comes with the fuzziness that occurs in the
lymph circulation at this season of the year, unless those precautions are taken and there is not the activity in those things with
which the body works at times, to which the body becomes allergic . . . These allergies come from an irritation to the superficial
circulation and lack of coordination of these with the alimentary
canal.   1541-12

In the present the blood supply, while very good, is—through the
lymph circulation—acting as an irritant to the soft tissue of nasal
passages. Hence the throat and eyes suffer because of too great a
flow of lymph, and the excitement apparent in the olfactory nerves
of the face and head tissue.
   These, as generally termed, are subject to inflammation by conditions to which the body becomes allergic at certain seasons or
cycles of body change; these produce a great irritation.   3180-1

Nervous system imbalance can also be a primary or contributing
factor in the development of allergies:

The pathological effect is being created by the reflex or sympathetic conditions in the functioning, or lack of functioning and coordination, of the cerebrospinal, sympathetic and vegetative with
sensory organisms.   5196-1

   . . . a self-consciousness of the lymph patches or spots where

there is connection or association with centers along the cerebrospinal system.   3224-1

Regardless of the cause–and–effect sequence, allergy symptoms can
be viewed as excessive reactions to irritants by a body in a weakened
state:

Q. Am I allergic to dust, and does it cause my colds?
A. Who isn't? All of these are just part of the general debilitation—
the inability of the circulation, because of these disturbances, to
call into play, as it were, sufficient of the leucocytes to destroy
dust. Or any sufficiently strong odors are just as harmful to the
body as dust.   3644-1

But this is the association more than it is the organic condition.
However, it can be just as severe as if the body sticks its nose in
the dust barrel or dust can! For, these are disturbances in the sensory system and in the glands of the body.   3556-1

While the majority of allergies in the readings were regarded as
physical in nature, a good number were partially, or even mostly, psychological. Consider Cayce's responses to the parents of two asthmatic
children:

Q. Is there any particular thing to which he is allergic?
A. Mostly to himself and his family!   2755-2

. . . and thus the body apparently becomes allergic to many of the
conditions about the body, but it is just as allergic to a suggestion
as it is to types of food.   5292-1

Without downplaying the seriousness of the symptoms or the importance of physical treatments, the readings go to great lengths to ensure that psychological aspects are also considered:

Q. Am I allergic to certain foods?

A. If you can imagine it, you can be allergic to most anything, if you want to!   3268-2

Q. Is there such a thing as allergy?
A. This is rather a fad. To be sure individuals may become allergic to certain conditions because of excess of certain elements in the body. But these are rather exaggerated oft.   3172-2

Q. Is any of this trouble due to allergy?
A. Some of it is due to allergy, but what is allergy? These are the effects of the imagination upon any influences that may react upon the olfactory or the sympathetic nerves.   3400-2

Q. Am I allergic to any substances?
A. Did you ever consider what is meant by being allergic? Most of it is in your imagination! Do you imagine things? Then you are allergic to it.   3586-1

There are pathological conditions, but there is more psychological. Psychological doesn't mean that the body is crazy, by any means, but has set ideas.   5211-1

Of the variety of recommendations for individuals with allergies, many of those found in the readings are indirect. Their purpose is to strengthen, cleanse, and coordinate body systems so any irritants in the diet or environment will simply be—less irritating. Known allergens should, of course, be avoided during this critical time with the understanding that this might not be necessary down the road.

The first order of business is often to speed the removal of toxins and congestion from the intestinal system. The importance of internal cleansing measures cannot be overestimated:

If we will cleanse the system, as we find, we should bring better conditions.   3400-2

There needs to be better coordination in eliminations.   1541-12

There are some pollens and odors (more odors with this body)
that are offensive, and thus the body is allergic to them. But these
also will disappear if there is better circulation created and if the
poisons are eliminated from the system.   3586-1

The types of internal cleansing measures mentioned include enemas,
colonics, mineral preparations like Eno salts, herbal preparations such
as ragweed and tonic formulas, and abdominal castor oil packs. In close
concert with these is an effort to sweeten the digestion and in some
cases soothe irritated intestinal walls. Supporting an alkaline, easily digested diet are prescriptions such as saffron tea, mullein tea, elm water,
and pepsin.

As would be expected, corrective dietary measures are an important
aspect of treatment. Typical instructions emphasize green vegetables,
fresh juices, yellow foods, meat juices, and the lighter proteins. Most
warnings concern meat fats, fried foods, sweets, starches, beer, and raw
apples. Specific combinations, such as seafood with sweets or acidic
foods, are sometimes vetoed as well.

Another frequent recommendation is osteopathic manipulation to
improve the flow of nerve impulses and, in some cases, correct extremely long–standing imbalances. Spinal realignment boosts the circulation and also helps the channels of elimination to work more smoothly:

These will relieve—if the adjustments are given to set up better
drainages.   1541-12

To reduce respiratory system congestion and promote expectoration,
an alcohol-based inhalant is often helpful. Glyco-Thymoline and the
Ray's products are advised as topical applications. Massage, hydrotherapy, and electrotherapy are part of many treatments.

A number of comments addressed allergy injections, which promote
desensitization by introducing tiny amounts of the offending substance
into the system. These were found to be sometimes helpful, sometimes
harmful, and usually avoidable:

To be sure, there may be given those elements hypodermically

that will react upon the body, but common reasoning should indicate that such is not as effective as would be nature's reproduc-
tion of itself in the body-forces . . . Of course, if it is the desire to
try to take shortcuts and you are too lazy to work, then do it!

3224-2

Q. Are the injections necessary this year to relieve hay fever?
A. This could be said, yes, and it could be said, no . . . It is not
necessary if following through or if the period is spent in some
other environ.
Q. When will the hay fever condition pass so no further injection
will be necessary?
A. This again depends upon how these are carried through and
where they are carried through. For if there is built the body-con-
sciousness that nothing else will do—nothing will do!   3436-3

We find that there are better ways than the administration of hypo-
dermics. These are good at times. But why put more poison as to
set up other conditions that later will be hard to combat, when
there has been caused—as it would in this body if kept up—disturbance . . . in the abdominal as well as lung area.   3556-1

Finally, the helpfulness of positive suggestion and a constructive attitude cannot be overemphasized:

And know they will not affect you, unless you let them!   386-3

Keep the right attitude, and do keep sweet.   1541-12

With the continuing of those things that attune the body to nature,
and the suggestions that attune the body to truth, to consciousness, we will break down the allergies . . .   3125-2

Do these and we will correct these conditions. But let the change
begin primarily in the mental attitude. . . . If the body continues to
worry over conditions that have arisen or that may arise, this will

prevent any of the applications from helping . . .   3556-1

The overriding message here is one of hope and promise. Freedom from allergies is within our grasp. Is it time to adopt a cat yet?

Hypochondria: When It IS All in the Mind

We can always find people (surely not us) who seem inclined to exaggerate, or even manufacture, alarming physical symptoms. Sometimes it is easy to see the stage being set for a crisis as fear, anxiety, confusion, or overly suggestible tendencies begin to get out of hand.

As the Cayce readings urge, each of us must come to acknowledge the part we play in our own state of health and learn how to take charge. The role of attitudes and emotions in illness is embodied in terms like "psychosomatic," which suggest this connection. Symptoms are at times thought to ease through the power of the placebo effect, which seems to work its magic through belief that a given treatment will do the trick.

To make some sense of this mind–over–matter mechanism, hypochondria and tendencies in that direction are touched on in advice given to twenty–three individuals. Although there were usually some real physical issues to be addressed as well, all of these people were told that their condition was at least partly psychological:

The *worry* of conditions produces the greater distresses with this body.   1000-5

What is it that you haven't got, if you set yourself to look for it!
                                                             3324-1

To be sure, there can be and at times there is, such anxiety about the general conditions and the reflexes that this brings on the very conditions which one fears.   5233-1

Mental . . . He has lost confidence in himself . . . We suggest to this man that he has a trouble with any organ of the system, and we will have that condition at times, in the system.   87-2

. . . one that assumes (or hypochondriac) . . . all those elements
that may be described by another.   2370-1

Although hypochondriac tendencies themselves are not usually attributed to physical causes, several seem closely associated in the readings. One is a duo of conditions known in Cayce's time as asthenia and neurasthenia. Asthenia, also sometimes referred to as general debilitation, is a temporarily weakened state due to illness, injury, or extreme stress. Neurasthenia is a more persistent form involving nerve or "battery" depletion that would probably be defined today as chronic fatigue. In this condition the brain itself is affected through hypersensitivity or a tendency to exaggerate:

The mind is alright, if it will act. The condition of the mind is acted
on by the mental force into the brain in itself, producing the condition we have now, of the neurasthenic . . . The action of the nerve
force on the brain itself proper, and it thinks it is sicker than it is.
                                                        17-1

The general condition, as we find, may be described as one of
neurasthenia; or a neurasthenic hypochondriac. Hence the conditions change or alter very materially from time to time, and whatever has been or is impressionable to the mind and to the
surroundings soon becomes a portion of the disorder.   483-1

. . . when there are cellular disturbances, and the body physical
able to create through its own impulse various effects of the conditions, then we may find much disturbance that may be *easily*
relieved, or we may find disturbances that will be *hard* to relieve—
dependent upon the attitude the individual . . . takes towards such
conditions.   1000-1

Poor coordination between the cerebrospinal and sympathetic nervous systems often turns up in these readings as well. A link between hypochondria and an overly stimulated imagination certainly makes sense:

> Hence the sympathetic nerves through the imaginative or vegetative nerve system have been affected. So, the body becomes rather a hypochondriac, in that it accepts or rejects without any consideration as to whether it is reasonable or unreasonable.
>
> 3452-1

> While the body is in that condition of being a hypochondriac or imagining only, we find that the effects of the sympathetic nervous system are such as to magnify the disorders to the physical body.   3585-1

> Some have called the condition neurotic, and others have termed it a portion of that condition wherein the mental application takes on every ill of every nature at one time or another; for such does become a portion of the body's disorders, as also do those things that may be helpful to the body.   754-1

Another closely related factor in these cases is the presence of some type of dysfunctional psychological state. In the readings these include anxiety, melancholia (depression, today), a lack of confidence, extreme suggestibility, and dementia:

> In the *nerve system*, this we find an effect and a cause, as is indicated, and produces such a nature as to be at times neurotic in its nature; so that any activity that is viewed by the body that is of a nature as to affect the body becomes hypochondriacal in its reaction to the system.   383-1

> . . . the mental attitude has become almost in that state of feeling that the body has symptoms of what it hears disturbs others.
>
> 3412-1

As would be expected, Cayce's primary treatments for the hypochondria itself focus on attitude adjustment. However, adjustment of the spine is often recommended, as well, along with other types of non-invasive treatments that lead to an increased sense of well being, such as massage, fume baths, dietary improvements, electrotherapy for circulation, and sun exposure for depression. Internal measures such as herbal tonics are rarely advised, perhaps because of the risk of psychological dependency:

> We would not make medicinal applications for this body; for, as indicated from the mental reactions, these would become a portion of the body as dependent upon same . . .   825-1

Regardless of the genuine physical imbalances being treated, Cayce's advice is always to focus on positive rather than negative outcomes so that the body's abundant potential for healing can be purposefully directed. A case in point is that of a psychiatrist who was told that despite occasional aches and pains, her ability to direct her own healing (or otherwise) was the strongest factor in her makeup:

> For, with this body more than most bodies, as we find, a conscious effort on the part of the body may make for almost whatever type of reaction physically that might be desired for the body.
> True, there are physical conditions that at times make for some disturbance; yet when the body stops itself to analyze same the body-mental is capable of knowing and experiencing not only the cause but that which to the great measure may correct that physical condition.   444-2

Although this is an unusual degree of self-knowledge and control, Cayce's advice to all seeking healing may be described as relentlessly constructive thinking:

> Think in wholly constructive manner; that is, as this: There is creative in the system that which may meet the needs of the physical body in its everyday activity, and sufficient to store energy for the resuscitation of *used* forces. Make that known in self. As the mind

accepts a condition as being *positive,* it *acts* upon that condition, yet when negative forces are continually set before self, and expected—and the expectancy is as of such to make the reaction of such a nature as to *destroy,* then *negative* forces become the more active. *Necessary,* then, that the body—*any* body—keep the near normal of a constructive building in the mind; for *mind* is the Builder.   202-4

No mental condition, now—don't get that way!   369-11

Do not create for self the attitude that "Now I've got sinus trouble—Now I've got this trouble, that trouble or the other!" because you'll have it! and you'll become a hypochondriac, should these conditions continue! Know "I'm getting better." Know, "I will meet these conditions as they come about." Know, "I'm doing these in the proper way and manner, and it will come about!"   911-4

. . . and keep the mind active in *doing* something—for others.
1000-2

. . . continue . . . interesting self in definite subjects, for definite conditions, for definite results.   1000-3

Know, as has been given, then, that the strength, the power, the influence to meet *any* emergencies within thine experience are ever present, at thine own disposal, if thou wilt but hold to that of the divinity within self to meet all of these.   1000-12

Do the things that have been outlined. But change the mental attitude of the body first, and we will find there will be more of a universal consciousness rather than a physical consciousness.
3412-1

By our thoughts, we are building health or illness into our bodies every day. If an ailment can be psychosomatic, then we now know how to put the cure in motion!

Closing the Door to Spirit Possession

Possession—the word evokes campy images of demonic head spinning and pea green spray for those of us who remember *The Exorcist* all too well. The exaggerations make it easier to forget that psychic takeovers have been with us for a long time and the realities can be quite scary (or just distasteful) indeed. It's reassuring to find that over seventy Cayce readings address this subject in a straightforward and hopeful manner and that priestly rituals are not required!

To put it simply, the phenomenon of possession refers to the overshadowing of a person's consciousness by one or more discarnate, or non-embodied, beings:

Q. What is it exactly that assails me?
A. Outside influences. Disincarnate entities.   5221-1

Entities that like to take people over do not tend to wish us well, as is demonstrated in biblical references to unclean spirits or devils. Jesus is reported to have cast out quite a few, and life readings given for several individuals mention this.

Although the term "spirit attachment" is often substituted today, Cayce would probably have treated an attachment as an early or less severe manifestation that could lead to full-blown possession if not checked. Or, in his own words: " . . . An organic disturbance is merely a possession when it has reached the nth degree as to be possession." (845-4)

Some of the many readings indexed as possession tendencies explain how a gradual openness toward spirit attachment can develop in the psyche. In one case, certain attitudes and poses had created habits " . . . that are *almost*—or at times, and under or in certain environments, become—*possessions!*" (1106-1) Similarly, a 440-16 report suggests that leaks in the aura lead to attachment or possession by discarnate beings and that certain types of vibrations can expel the negative entities and seal the leaks.

A person's openness to this kind of takeover, therefore, always begins with a loss of conscious control, due to one or several factors. A

primary cause given in at least twenty–five readings is a lack of coordination between the cerebrospinal and autonomic nervous systems. In
such cases an injury or stress of some other origin causes a lesion or
subluxation to form, often in the lower spine. The resulting interference
with nerve impulses and glandular functions leads to chronic discomfort, depression, and an over–reliance on methods of dulling that pain.
Or, a "perfect storm" of nervous shock coupled with an unwitting openness to "psychic forces" might create a situation where: " . . . We have
possession here." (638–1)

Since chronic pain is so often treated chemically, it is easy to see how
there could be a strong link with alcoholism, a factor in at least eleven
cases of possession. Viewed in this light, when people who drink to
excess don't act like themselves, perhaps they aren't! It is the release of
control that makes a takeover possible:

Q. What causes him to lose control of himself?
A. Possession! . . .
Q. Does that mean by other entities, while under the influence of
liquor?
A. By others while under the influence that causes the reactions
and makes for the antagonism, and the very *change* of the activities.   1183-3

Whether possession occurs at such times may be dictated by the
choice to give way to strong physical appetites:

Not a possession, save when there begins the gratifying of same;
then there are the opportunities for those influences from without
to possess the activities of the body . . .   1439-1

It is evidently possible for a person to be taken over not only by
entities but also by the spirit of addictive substances:

. . . the condition has reached such as may be termed possessed
with the spirit of both rum *and* the sedatives to keep the satisfying
of these influences . . . and when *inordinate* desire has been cre-

ated by the use of those forces that make for the activities in all the sensory forces of the body, it becomes as the possession of those forces from without and from within that create, without the cleansing influence of the spiritual entering in from without, that which is hard to cope with.   486-1

The hazards of consciously inviting spirit possession by offering oneself as a medium become apparent in ten or more cases. These readings warn against approaches such as automatic writing, which could cause a psychic opening to occur without the proper safeguards in place. Those who have forced an awakening of the kundalini or life force energies within the body are especially vulnerable to spirits attracted by that flow. The result can be quite an energy drain:

Q. Are there entities, because of a psychic opening, feeding on or sucking my vitality?
A. Entities that would seek to find expression through that left open.   436-3

Mental illness is a closely related factor that can be found in an equal number of cases. Those who allow unseen beings to control them, whether under the influence or not, because of anger, depression, nervous breakdown, or full blown psychosis, can be viewed as not in their right mind by definition:

The mind, through anger, may make the body do that which is contrary to the better influences of same . . . Then, through pressure upon some portion of the anatomical structure that would make for the disengaging of the natural flow of the mental body through the physical in its relationships to the soul influence, one may be dispossessed of the mind; thus ye say rightly he is "out of his mind."   281-24

Q. Is he crazy, or mentally deranged?
A. If possession isn't crazy, what is it?   1183-3

Dementia, though attributed to a general weakening of body systems, can also create openness to "outside entities" simply because the mind is naturally becoming more in touch with their domain:

Such, then, become possessed as of hearing voices, because of their closeness to the Borderland. Many of these are termed deranged when they may have more of a closeness to the universal than one who may be standing nearby and commenting; yet they are awry when it comes to being normally balanced or healthy for their activity in a material world.   281-4

Glandular imbalance, cited in eight or more cases, is apparently a factor in many psychic openings. The second center, sometimes referred to as the "cells of Leydig," is centrally involved in conception and sometimes also in possession dynamics:

There has been the opening of the lyden (Leydig) gland and thus a disturbance through glandular system. Possession at times is the result.   3410-1

The risk of a hostile entity takeover is evidently also present in cases of epilepsy where blackouts occur during attacks:

Q. How may epileptics possessed by an unclean spirit be designated or be known?
A. As to whether there be consciousness or not *through* the falling or spell! Those that are unconscious are possessed, or are possessed during that unconsciousness—see?   281-4

Cayce's treatments for possession and tendencies in that direction always focus on correcting imbalances and strengthening areas of physical and psychological weakness. Typically this requires a three-pronged approach.

In at least half of these cases the first order of business is to properly align the spine in order to address physical discomfort at its source and promote normal functions in the brain and elsewhere:

> As we find . . . depossession may be made by the creating for a
> balance between the coordinating influences in the brain activity
> and responses . . .   638-1

Although osteopathic adjustments are most often indicated for this
purpose, both chiropractic and neuropathy also receive mention. Massage is similarly employed in eighteen cases, either as an alternative or
supporting treatment. On several occasions, use of an electric vibrator
is preferred " . . . so that the vibratory forces of the body are changed—
thus producing coordinations and the deflections of those influences
that disturb the body." (1572-1)

Another primary form of treatment, also found in about half of these
cases, is electrotherapy. As in the above reference, the purpose of all
types of electrical treatments is to change the very vibrations of the
body so as to make control by discarnate entities impossible. Although
actual modalities vary widely, the Violet Ray, Wet Cell, and Radio-Active Appliance receive the most frequent endorsement. Their purpose is
extremely consistent:

> . . . to *close* as it were the centers through the system to the influ-
> ences from without . . .   282-8

> These low electrical forces will aid in eliminating the tendencies
> for possession.   2865-1

> Hence the electrical forces will aid, with the suggestions, in elimi-
> nating these *impressions*—or *possessions* of the mental attitudes.
>   1553-6

Exceptions to electrotherapy are always made in cases of ongoing
alcohol consumption because using them close together is regarded as
extremely harmful. However, treatment following a period of abstinence
can be highly beneficial:

> For this body (the husband), if there could be a sufficient period of
> refraining from the use of alcoholic stimulants and the . . . electri-

cal treatments used these would drive the conditions out!
    But do not use same with the effects of alcohol in the system—
it would be detrimental!   1183-3

A third category of treatments approaches protection from a mental-spiritual perspective. One way to strengthen the resistance to unwanted influences is through positive, or even hypnotic, suggestion. The words are basically affirmations designed to remind the subject, in a non-directed way, of his or her spiritual nature. For those who are able, regular Bible reading is also strongly advised. Both are helpful means of " . . . awakening of forces within self that may combat evil influences in the inner life . . . " (486-1) Magnetic healing also receives occasional mention, as in the following vibration-raising method given specifically for those with epilepsy:

This may be accomplished by placing the left hand over the abdominal region and the right hand over the 9th and 10th dorsal or solar plexus ganglia, and so held for half to three-quarters of an hour each day. It will leave!   281-4

Many additional treatments, including hydrotherapy, diet, packs, sedatives, and various other types of prescriptions, are found throughout these readings. Although all are intended to help the body regain its normal functions, there is only one direct reference to our topic. Cayce's comments on possession, alcoholism, and gold are quite intriguing:

Q. In alcoholic cases, can a general outline of treatment be given?
A. No. Each individual has its own individual problems. Not all are physical. Hence there are those that are of the sympathetic nature, or where there has been the possession by the very activity of same; but gold will destroy desire in any of them!   606-1

So, once again the readings leave us with plenty to ponder. The presence of disembodied spirits all around us is taken for granted. Helpful ones may well be attracted to persons consciously on the spiritual path, but there are always those that: " . . . May obsess *anyone* that opens self to listen to same!" (2067-3) Clearly we need to be careful out there. Spinning heads are best avoided at any time.

Breathing as a Way of Life

Few things are taken more for granted in life than breathing—until there's a hitch. Then we see where the true priority lies. The old joke where the sage consulted about the meaning of life responds with, "Keep breathing as long as possible" is right on. Human life on earth begins with the first breath, when the Cayce readings say the soul typically enters the body, and ends with the last, when it departs for higher realms. This connection between breath and spirit is abundant in our language in words like respiration, inspire, and perspire.

So we know that we must breathe to live, but how many of us make a conscious effort to improve the depth of our breathing, or even make a connection between breathing more fully and embracing life more abundantly? The readings confirm what yoga and breath work practitioners have always understood. Focusing on breath is important, and breathing exercises can be a vital key to wellness.

What's so healthy about breathing? To begin with, it's one way the body disposes of metabolic waste:

> Breath is the life-blood cleansing of the body, normally—see? For, there are the needs for the combination of the gases as inhaled to act upon the purifying of the system.   2072-5

Taking fuller breaths will facilitate this process and have an energizing effect:

> . . . be able to so exercise self as to get up a good perspiration; be able to so function that in the throwing off of refuses from the system, the respiratory system will act, and a breath may be taken—*good, full, deep*—into the lungs, and the activity and buoyancy of life itself, as is gathered from all forces about it, must radiate through the system . . .   412-1

Dr. Harold Reilly gives a more detailed explanation of how and why this works:

A great deal of elimination takes place through the lungs, by means of deep breathing. When you take a good deep breath, especially if you exhale it completely, forcing the residual air out of the lungs, you bring about a complete change of air. By doing so, you not only drive oxygen down into the lower part of the lungs, but you also help to speed the elimination of carbon dioxide, which is the end product of fatigue. Protein waste is also eliminated through the lungs in the form of carbon dioxide. The bloodstream picks up some of the acid waste and turns it into gas, which is exchanged for oxygen in the lungs.[43]

For the most part, Reilly, Cayce, and the time-honored discipline of yoga take a similar exercise-oriented approach toward deep breathing routines. These are ideally to take place either outdoors or near an open window with the body free of restrictive clothing:

The breathing exercises night and morning would be taken in this manner:
   Stand before an open window, or where there is good, fresh air. Use the arms, the upper portion of the body, the head, the neck exercises; taking two or three movements in each activity; rising on the feet with the arms gently stretched above the head, breathing in deep through the nostrils, and breathing out through the mouth, in each of these activities; circling the head and neck, and some bending exercise of the body.   1787-4

Well that there be an exercise morning and evening. Of evenings, the exercise would be rather that of the lower limbs; while of morning, just before dressing—after bathing, or before bathing—exer-

[43]Harold J. Reilly and Ruth Hagy Brod, *The Edgar Cayce Handbook for Health Through Drugless Therapy* (New York: Macmillan Publishing Co., Inc., 1975), 33.

cise *above* the waist, of the circular motion of the head and neck, raising and lowering of the arms, swinging these back and forward, that we may *expand* the chest and raising on feet with the lifting of the chest, with deep breath—inhalation and exhalation.

427-4

Done over time, as these exercises improve the body's circulation and balance, they will lead to a greater sense of wellness:

Hence if there will be morning and evening the exercise, not the stooping but the bending—raising the hands high above the head—as these are slowly raised, rising on toes, drawing *in* the deep breath through the nostril—as the body is bent forward, with the fingers toward the floor, exhale through the mouth—doing this *slowly*, consistently, for a minute or such, morning and evening— we may find conditions on the mend.   257-172

For these as the body will find will tend to make for, morning and evening, the throwing off of refuse as it were from the throat and head and the bronchial tubes. And with the exercises in the open, as recuperative forces at play and at work, will make for the more helpful and the more enlivening of the whole of the body-physical forces.   257-173

Such an exercise would be that described as the *stretching* of the arms, the lower limbs, with the intake and the sudden exhale from the lungs themselves; that not only purifies the activity of the source of energizing—or the energies for the blood supply—but alleviates those tendencies for the pressures that are indicated in the cervical areas.   989-1

As this last and other excerpts show, spinal pressures can sometimes interfere with the ability to take full breaths, although deep breathing itself may sometimes relieve this. To be on the safe side, it is best to have the spine checked if breathing becomes impaired and before engaging in new exercise programs.

Precautions also apply to breathing routines alone, which have huge therapeutic and even transpersonal potential, but must be carefully tailored to individual readiness. Regarding this potential, Cayce remarked:

> There may be set a mode of circulation through the breathing exercises for almost any type of condition, see . . .   288-40

However, this does not mean that everyone will benefit from the same exercises. An individual who was questioning the value of a breath–holding procedure endorsed by the Rosicrucians was told:

> To this body, as we find, this would be rather strenuous. If the body were one that took more violent exercise, physically, it might not be bad. But the greater exercise of the body here is of the *mental* self.   816-12

A more in-depth response was given to a practitioner of alternate breathing and cleansing breath who asked for an explanation of the use of breathing and its purifying qualities. Cayce began by advising that these exercises be curtailed until the general health had improved:

> These are well when there are *not* physical hindrances to their more perfect activity. That help has been obtained when there are already obstructions indicates the greater benefit that might be had *if* there were the normal flow of impulse from glands and nerve centers raised by activities of breathing.   2072-5

The reading went on to outline a gentler approach of inhaling deeply through the right nostril and holding it as long as possible while gradually rising on the toes, raising the arms so more air could enter the chest, then exhaling sharply through the mouth. After at least three repetitions and a short rest, this sequence would be repeated with the left nostril, adding a slow turn to the left from the waist while rising on the toes. Later on, after spinal corrections had been made, these exercises could be " . . . altered by *direction* of breath—as well as position of body." (2072-5)

But the most detailed information on breathing was given to a person who had been experimenting with yogic breathing and meditation. Cayce found the practice itself excellent but far too powerful to be taken so lightly:

> For, *breath* is the basis of the living organism's activity. Thus, such exercises may be beneficial or detrimental in their effect upon a body.   2475-1

By detrimental effects he is referring to raising kundalini energy without the proper safeguards, which might be likened to lion taming for amateurs:

> As has been experienced, this opening of the centers or the raising of the life force may be brought about by certain characters of breathing—for, as indicated, the breath is power in itself; and this power may be directed to certain portions of the body. But for what purpose? As yet it has been only to see what will happen! Remember what curiosity did to the cat!   2475-1

This person was strongly counseled to slow down, purify himself mentally and physically, and consciously formulate a spiritual ideal. Then, he could proceed:

> By all means! If and when, and *only* when, preparation has been made; and when there is the knowledge, the understanding and the wisdom as to what to do *with* that gained! Without such, do not undertake same!   2475-1

Under the right conditions, breathing as a devotional exercise has much to teach us, as Cayce and others attest:

> When we breathe, we fill our bodies with this vital energy. To inhale is to breathe in the spirit of God, to take in life itself. Our breath is the connecting link between the life force and the physical body, and breathing for the purpose of expanding our aware-

ness connects us naturally to the Divine within . . . It brings . . . expanded awareness, compassion and vitality to the very depths of our being.[44]

Let us all inspire each other to inhale more deeply and embrace the divinity in life.

Keys to Rejuvenescence

We all know by now that diet and lifestyle choices influence both how and how quickly we age. One result of studies on this topic is ample confirmation of the Cayce material on various aspects of what we might call preventive health care.

Slowing the signs of aging is a worthy goal, but is it possible to go a step or two further and stop the clock, or even reverse the process? To this question the readings give an emphatic yes!

Such a radical possibility goes way beyond common catch phrases such as "anti-aging." The readings favor the term rejuvenation for the process by which entire bodies, or certain systems, are made youthful again. Rejuvenation, according to the dictionary, creates a state of rejuvenescence, a delightful word for growing young.

Clues to the attainment of rejuvenescence are found throughout both the physical and life readings. An entire reading that focuses on rejuvenation comments that maintaining one's health in the first place is the more natural (and attractive!) course, but a body can, indeed, be revitalized with the right proactive approach:

The better manner, to be sure is the *preservation*—which is not only as a first law but is the more comely in its application. To be sure, as it has been indicated again and again, there is that within the physical forces of the body—if it is kept in a constructive way and manner—which may be revivified or rejuvenated . . . This requires, necessarily, the proper thinking, the proper living, the

---

[44]Kathleen Barratt, *Dance of Breath* (self-published, 1993), 37.

proper application of those influences in the experience of an *entity* in its associations with everything about a body.　　681-2

Many of the specifics unfold in the course of the above reading and others. When asked for an ideal diet, Cayce offers broad guidelines intended to take changing needs into account:

There might be one diet given today and then next week you would have another! That which keeps the spittle or salivary reaction alkaline. That which keeps the blood reaction, by test, negative. That which keeps the urine eliminations as a balance at twenty-four . . . without albumin, without sediment, and with an alkaline tendency; but not too great a tendency. That which makes for the proper eliminations and body-building without becoming superfluous flesh, or drainage to same—see? Hence these are to be kept by *constructive* measures and forces, see?　　681-2

Exercise instructions are given in broad strokes as well:

No better exercises may be taken than the stretching exercise; as rising on toes—and this doesn't mean with shoes on!—on heels, rocking back and forth; stretching the arms upward, the bending exercises, what may be literally termed . . . the cat-stretching exercises, which includes, of course, being able—(put very coarsely)—to do the split, be able to put the head on the feet, to put the feet behind the head, to make the head and neck exercises . . . To be sure, in the present . . . conditions that exist, must be gone at gently; but be persistent morning and evening, working at it, still not letting it become rote, but purposeful.　　681-2

Also mentioned in this and many other readings is the nerve rejuvenating influence of the Radio–Active Appliance:

. . . adding to the system those vibrations as would be found in the activity of the Radio-Active Appliance carrying into the system those vibrations that will *create* for the system the rejuvenation of

the impulses through the gray active forces of the nerve impulse
itself.   241-1

Using this device with gold makes it an aid to cellular renewal as
well as for " . . . stimulation to the gland functioning and to the rejuvenation of the cell *building* centers that are built within the division of
blood cell in spleen, brain, and in the *lacteal ducts* . . . " (200–1)
This principle of vibration is also employed with other types of electrotherapy for rejuvenating effects:

And the activities of the violet ray are only to make for the electrical rejuvenation of nerve energies that have been depleted through
the inactivity of the whole system of this body.   676-1

But this continual vibration as set here by the application of the
electrically driven vibrator . . . will bring about a rejuvenation of
the nerve centers in such a way as to supply new life, as it were, to
the organs of the body.   3721-1

. . . the body would be treated with the ultra violet Ray to produce
rejuvenation of all the Lymphatic forces and give resistance to the
body.   3724-1

Regular spinal manipulation, often advised to restore the body's
proper energy flow, is regarded as complementary to electrical treatments:

For in the applying of the electrical vibration, these are necessarily rejuvenating the electrical forces of the body as is related to
nerve energy of the system. While the manipulations, properly
given, are to apply to that direction through which the rejuvenation of energy is directed, see?   5536-5

This complementary nature is also true of the invigorating effects of
massage and seaside rest cures:

232 Edgar Cayce's Everyday Health

The better would be sun, salt, and sand, and these—with gentle massage at or after such sand, sun and salt water baths—would bring the rejuvenation to the nerves, and build up the blood supply. 71-1

Breathing fresh air, in particular, is noted as having an enlivening effect on the blood:

The more air or oxygen, the quicker will be the proper rejuvenation of the blood supply. 428-3

Herbal tonics that cleanse and revitalize the system can be equally energizing in their effect:

Thus aiding the whole system in its *rejuvenation,* as related to the effect of *drosses* in the physical body. 5509-3

Measures such as these are all essential pieces of the puzzle when it comes to keeping our batteries properly charged. The trick is to use them in a constructive plan to keep all body functions in harmony with each other:

The body must see, to be rejuvenated, the body must be kept in a condition of construction; to ever find that the heart, the digestive organs' combination, the elimination and assimilation, the hair, the scalp, the nasal, the eye, the ear, the throat, the bronchi, the lungs, the structural forces of the body work as a *unit*—or as *one!* And then we may find, and do find, the body *building,* ever. 681-2

The resulting youthful glow is just what the doctor ordered so long as beauty is not sought as an end in itself but is shared with others for a higher purpose:

[Be] . . . not only physically fit for beauty but physically fit for the beauties of self—soul—development as it may apply to helpful,

hopeful things, conditions, experiences that may be brought in to
the experience of others.   681-2

This leads us to another dimension of renewal that is less discussed
because it is metaphysical in nature. Several individuals were told in
their readings that they could heal or recharge themselves through a
combination of visualization, intention, and spiritual attunement exercises:

> . . . if the body will see, feel, know in self there is being enacted in
> self that which brings life's resuscitation in the earth, there may be
> felt that rejuvenation that only comes with the closer walk and
> communion with Him . . .   326-3

One of these talented individuals was Edgar Cayce himself, who, in
an early Egyptian lifetime, had reportedly succeeded in rejuvenating
his body at an advanced age. Although the priest Ra-Ta may well have
practiced certain physical disciplines, life readings on the subject do not
focus on this at all. Instead they emphasize meditation, prayer, releasing
stressful emotions, refraining from negativity, and devotion to a life of
service:

> . . . there were the needs for the Priest to enter into that period of
> meditation, of setting himself aside, purifying through continuous
> prayer, continuous seeking, continuous opening of those forces
> . . . Thus we had the Priest's rejuvenation, or the turning back of
> age as it were, or those conditions which would hinder the activi-
> ties.   281-43

> . . . the regeneration of the body came to him through the casting
> aside, as it were, of the years of toil and strife through which the
> body of Ra-Ta itself had passed . . .   696-1

With the return then of the priest to the Temple Beautiful, there
first began the priest to withdraw himself from the whole that regeneration in body might become manifest, and the body lay down
the material weaknesses—and from those sources of regeneration

recreated the body in its *elemental* forces . . .   294-150

The priest in body . . . in the height of the development was at the regeneration, or when over a hundred years . . . in the earth.
275-38

Anyone who thinks he's too old to start the rejuvenescence process rolling had better think again!

A Prescription for Healthy Living

Cayce's health advice always seems so spot-on that it's only natural to speculate about what one's own reading might have been like. Not that there is any shortage of professional psychics in the Virginia Beach area. But for many, the readings are still the best resource, especially when it comes to wellness. That's why they have been consulted at length in compiling the following ten-point set of healthy living instructions. Each was mentioned hundreds of times with enough variations and special considerations to fill a book, so please consider this a very brief introduction. And remember—once a prescription has been obtained, the real challenge is to do what it says!

Eat Whole Foods

. . . the body *{should}* keep that diet for the system that the physical needs through its inmost desires, and not override those conditions by the will of the individual."   257-6

Conflicting studies and changing fads make this topic seem complicated when the real trick here is discovering one's own ideal menu plan and then mustering the self discipline to follow it. The central step in this process is to avoid junk, which actually disguises our inmost cravings, and instead consume a wide variety of real foods. Feel free to vary the menu as inspiration strikes, so long as it consists of fresh produce, whole grains, eggs, nuts, fish, moderate meat, and so forth. At the same time give all refined products (white bread, pasta, rice, sugar) a pass. Cravings will actually start to shift.

Drink Plenty of Water

Do drink more water.   2051-7

According to a multitude of sources, most of us may well be dehydrated much of the time. An important book titled *Your Body's Many Cries for Water* points out numerous links between chronic dehydration and common disorders.[45] Of course, all liquids help us stay hydrated, but water is unique in its capacity to flush the kidneys and intestinal tract. That's why it's best to drink six to eight glasses daily, between meals, starting with half a glassful of lukewarm water upon arising.

Exercise Every Day

To be sure, the body should take as much physical exercise—and in the open—as is practical each day, not to be overstrenuous.
                                                                   2153-4

Due to a variety of factors, most people suffer from exercise deficit rather than the reverse. The best way to remedy this, where possible, is to start walking every day. Besides providing the benefits of fresh air and moderate sunlight, those daily strides tone and strengthen muscles, stimulate the heart, relax the nerves, and even promote digestion. Other healthy choices include stretches, rotations, swimming, bicycle riding, yoga, sports, and games.

Get Enough Rest

Also the *{healing}* response depends greatly on whether or not there is the opportunity given for rest . . .   902-1

---

[45]F. Batmanghelidj, *Your Body's Many Cries for Water* (Virginia: Global Health Solutions, Inc., 2001).

Whether we receive as much sleep as we need can make the difference between sickness and health, as everyone who has pushed the envelope too far and caught a cold knows. The body sends out sleepiness signals when it needs to recharge. All we need to do is obey, whenever that is humanly possible. Sometimes it's helpful to promote nighttime relaxation with a warm bath, gentle stretching, a back rub, or a soothing cup of herbal tea.

Cleanse That Colon

For, *every* one—everybody—should take an internal bath occasionally, as well as an external one. They would all be better off if they would!   440-2

The condition of the large intestine serves as a health indicator for the rest of the body. In fact, Cayce saw many health problems as originating with constipation, blockages, and toxic buildup in this area before colon cancer was even in the news. Easy ways to promote colon health include dietary fiber, a high water intake, occasional fruit fasts, short-term laxative use as well as enemas and colonic irrigations.

Keep the Spine Aligned

But if there is the persistency, we will find we may be able to remove those inclinations for the lack of coordination in the nerve reflexes . . .   1476-2

Nerve impulses originating in the spinal cord travel to virtually every part of the body, so it's important to keep the pathways they move on clear. Chiropractic and osteopathy offer time honored methods of lining up the vertebrae so circulation can flow freely. Injury and stress are common causes of misalignments, so chronic discomfort can be our guide as to when to get checked.

Receive Regular Massage

> This will not only keep a stimulating . . . but will aid in keeping the
> body beautiful . . .   1968-7

There's nothing quite like massage for toning muscles, relaxing nerves, and promoting blood and lymph circulation. In fact, it affects the body much like exercise, with the added benefits of skin replenishing oils and positive touch. Professional body work is always therapeutic but sometimes a back or foot rub from a friend or family member is all that is needed.

Practice Positive Thinking

> To be sure, the attitudes oft influence the physical condition of the
> body.   4021-1

Often quoted phrases like "mind is the builder" and "thoughts are things" urge us to consider the impact of our attitudes—toward ourselves, those around us, and life in general. Positive thinking requires a conscious intent and some inspiration through sources such as reading, humor, service opportunities, worship, study groups, music, prayer, and work with ideals.

Center the Mind

> The body mental and spiritual needs spiritual food—prayer, medi-
> tation, thinking upon spiritual things.   4008-1

Learning how to still the mind and center it on an ideal is part of reaching our full potential as human beings. It is only by pushing the pause button that the still small voice of Spirit can be heard. One of the many healthy side effects of meditation, prayer, and spiritual study is an improved control of tension-producing emotions.

Remember Some Dreams

Sleep—that period of time when the soul takes stock of that it has acted upon during one rest period to another . . .   5754-2

All who sleep engage in dreaming, whether their content is recalled in the morning or not. It's helpful to be familiar with the concerns that occupy us at unconscious levels for a variety of reasons, including the chance of spotting important clues to health. The best way to stimulate dream recall is to express the conscious intent, remain still on awakening, and make a note of whatever is brought back, no matter how silly or embarrassing it seems.

Renew this Prescription Indefinitely

This is actually an eleventh point. Enough said!

Bibliography

An Edgar Cayce Home Medicine Guide. Virginia: A.R.E. Press, 1986.

Balch, James F., and Phyllis A. Balch. *Prescription for Nutritional Healing.* New York: Avery Publishing Group, 1997.

Baraff, Carol A. *The Atomidine Story.* Virginia: Heritage Publications, 1978.

Barratt, Kathleen. *Dance of Breath.* Self-published, 1993.

Batmanghelidj, F. *Your Body's Many Cries for Water.* Virginia: Global Health Solutions, Inc., 2001.

Cayce, Edgar Evans. *Two Electrical Appliances Described in the Edgar Cayce Readings.* Virginia: A.R.E. Press, 1972.

Cigales, M., T. Field, B. Lundy, A. Cuadra, and S. Hart. "Massage Enhances Recovery from Habituation in Normal Infants." *Infant Behavior and Development* (January 1997): 29–34.

Cuomo, Rosario, Rafella Grasso, Giovanni Sarnelli, Gaetano Capuano, Emanuele Nicolai, Gerardo Nardone, Domenico Pomponi, Gabriele Budillon, and Enzo Ierardi. "Effects of Carbonated Water on Functional Dyspepsia and Constipation." *European Journal of Gastroenterology & Hepatology* (September 2002): 991–99.

Davis, Paul, and Christine Iwahashi. "Whole Almonds and Almond Fractions Reduce Aberrant Crypt Foci in a Rat Model of Colon Carcinogenesis." *Cancer Letter* (April 2001): 27–33.

Field, T., S. Schanberg, M. Davalos, and J. Malphurs. "Massage with Oil Has More Positive Effects on Normal Infants." *Pre and Perinatal Psychology Journal* (Winter 1996): 75–80.

Hu, F.B., and M.J. Stampfer. "Nut Consumption and Risk of Coronary Heart Disease: A Review of Epidemiologic Evidence." *Current Atherosclerosis Reports* (November 1999): 204–9.

Joseph, James A., Barbara Shukitt-Hale, Natalia A. Denisova, Donna Bielinski, Antonio Martin, John J. McEwen, and Paula C. Bickford. "Reversals of Age-Related Declines in Neuronal Signal Transduction, Cognitive, and Motor Behavioral Deficits with Blueberry, Spinach, or Strawberry Supplementation." *The Journal of Neuroscience* (September 15, 1999): 19 (18): 8114–121.

Kilham, Chris. "Coffee and Chocolate, the New Health Foods." *HerbalGram* 47 (Fall 1999): 21.

Kris-Etherton, P.M., S. Yu-Poth, J. Sabate, H.E. Ratcliffe, G. Zhao, and T.D. Etherton. "Nuts and their Bioactive Constituents: Effects on Serum Lipids and Other Factors that Affect Disease Risk." *American Journal of Clinical Nutrition* (September 1999): 504–11.

McGarey, William A. and Associated Physicians of the A.R.E. Clinic. *The Physician's Reference Notebook.* Virginia: A.R.E. Press, 1996.

Mora, S., I–M Lee, J.E. Buring, and P.M. Ridker. "Association of Physical Activity and Body Mass Index with Novel and Traditional Cardiovascular Biomarkers in Women." *Journal of the American Medical Association* (March 2006): 1412–19.

Ott, John. *Health and Light: the Effects of Natural and Artificial Light on Man and Other Living Things.* Old Greenwich, Connecticut: Devin–Adair Publishing, 1972.

Owen, R.W., A. Giacose, W.E. Hull, R. Haubner, G. Wurtele, B. Spiegelhalder, and H. Bartsch. "Olive–Oil Consumption and Health: The Possible Role of Antioxidants." *The Lancet Oncology* (October 2000): 107–12.

Reilly, Harold J. and Ruth Hagy Brod. *The Edgar Cayce Handbook for Health Through Drugless Therapy.* New York: Macmillan Publishing Co., Inc., 1975.

Scafidi, F.A., T.M. Field, S.M. Schanberg, C.R. Bauer, K. Tucci, J. Roberts, C. Morrow, and C.M. Kuhn. "Massage Stimulates Growth in Preterm Infants: A Replication." *Infant Behavior and Development* (April–June 1990): 167–88.

Schulze, Richard. *25 Ways to Have the Cleanest Kidneys.* California: Natural Healing Publications, 2004.

———. *Dr. Schulze's 2011 Herbal Product Catalog.* Marina Del Rey, CA: American Botanical Pharmacy, 2011.

———. *Healing Liver and Gallbladder Disease Naturally.* California: Natural Healing Publications, 2003.

Spiller, Gene A., David A.J. Jenkins, Ottavio Bosello, Joan E. Gates, Liz N.

Cragen, and Bonnie Bruce. "Nuts and Plasma Lipids: An Almond-Based Diet Lowers LDL-C while Preserving HDL-C." *Journal of the American College of Nutrition* (June 1998): 285–90.

Steward, H. Leighton, Morrison C. Bethea, Sam S. Andrews, and Luis A. Balart. *The New Sugar Busters!* New York: Ballantine Books, 2003.

Toda Y., S. Takemura, T. Morimoto, and R. Ogawa. "Relationship between HLA-DRB1 genotypes and efficacy or oral type II collagen treatment using chicken cartilage soup in rheumatoid arthritis." *Nihon Rinsho Meneki Gakkai Kaishi* (February, 1997): 44–51.

Weil, Andrew. *Spontaneous Healing.* New York: Alfred A. Knopf, 1995.

Wigley, Fredrick M. "Exercise after 50 Can Add Three Years to Life Expectancy." *Duke Medicine Health News* (January 2006): 2.

About the Author

Carol A. Baraff is a massage therapist and long-time researcher and author of publications inspired by the Edgar Cayce readings, particularly those associated with holistic health and practical application of natural remedies. After living near the Association for Research and Enlightenment (A.R.E.) in Virginia Beach, VA for most of the past forty-one years, she has recently relocated to the southwestern part of the state, just down the road from the A.R.E. Camp.

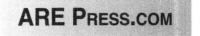